BREAST CANCER

From Diagnosis to Surgery

By

Dr. Charley Ferrer

Publisher
Cancer Tamer, Inc.
PO Box 60985
Staten Island NY 10306
info@cancerTamer.org
718-916-4124

Print: 978-0-9982202-0-8
Digital: 978-0-9982202-1-5

Printing: May & June 2017

Library of Congress Catalog Card Number: Pending

Cover Photo: Scott Church
Cover Design & Print Book Formatting
Cynthia Arsuaga, I Heart Books
Proofread and e-Book Formatting
Concierge Self-Publishing

The views and opinions provided in this book are not intended as medical advice. They are merely one women's experience with breast cancer. Always consult with your medical provider(s) for the treatment that is best for you. This book is written from the perspective of breast cancer; however, it can be used for any type of cancer whether you're a woman, man or child.

www.CancerTamer.org

Dedicated to the *Cancer Tamer* in **YOU**
because you shouldn't be at war
with your body!

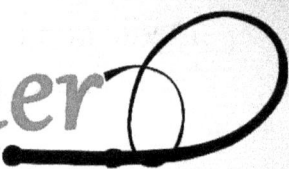

Cancer Tamer

because you shouldn't be at war with your body!

Cancer Tamer Philosophy & Mission

For decades, we've been taught to fight, overcome and survive the war against cancer. We have forgotten that cancer is not an "outside force" invading but an "inside force" residing. It's in our breast, our blood, our DNA; and in our attempts to destroy it, we inadvertently destroy ourselves.

I believe that if we discover how to "tame" the cancer within through exercise, nutrition, holistic approaches, self-empowerment and more, we'll live longer, happier, more fulfilling lives.

Cancer Tamer is dedicated to empowering women and creating new products and services to achieve that goal. We provide workshops on how to deal with cancer and the obstacles you'll face. We also created workshops for physicians and health-care providers to remind them that women are more than just their tumor diagnosis.

Cancer Tamer also hosts a special Body Love Retreat for women to help them reconnect with their bodies and their sensual essence — something which is all too often overlooked and lost during this phase of our lives.

Our goal is to empower women! That is why this 3-part book series on breast cancer was created; as was the Cancer Tamer Television Talk Show which you can view on our website or YouTube. Plus, we've collaborated with several sponsors to provide our members with FREE or discounted services not readily available elsewhere. Thus, sign-up for our newsletter today and become part of the *Cancer Tamer* movement and empower your life!

Contents

FOREWORD

Dr. Charley Ferrer

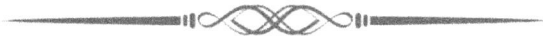

Being diagnosed with breast cancer is scary.

Let me rephrase that, it's terrifying as hell!

It's the closest thing to walking to the executioner's block and seeing the sun shine off his sharpened axe, imagining your blood already dripping from it. Or being made to walk the plank in shark-infested waters only to glance at the sea below and discover Jaws is there waiting for you, licking his razor-sharp teeth as he anticipates his next meal.

I recall standing before my bathroom sink, staring into the mirror and whispering, "You're sick, Charley." I felt something was wrong with me — I'd sensed it for months. My friends reassured me that I was fine, and my symptoms were merely stress-related as I was putting in 16- to 18-hour days to promote my business and the conferences and workshops I conduct. It wasn't until December 18, 2015 that the thought crossed my mind to perform a breast self-exam; after all, it had been months, perhaps a year or so since I'd done one. That's when I discovered the lump in my right breast.

Since I worked for myself and couldn't afford health insurance, I often told myself, "You're not allowed to get sick." I trusted my body to listen. Okay, I'll concede that's not the greatest logic, but it did work for me for years. At least, I thought it did.

It wasn't until February 1, 2016, over 43 days after discovering the lump, that my new health insurance kicked in, and I was able to see a physician. That physician immediately referred me for a mammogram with contrast and an ultrasound of my breasts in addition to performing a full battery of blood tests.

The mammogram and ultrasound both detected a large undifferentiated mass in my right breast measuring over 3.9

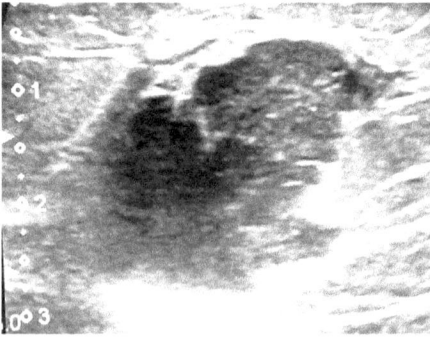

centimeters. As I sat there and stared at the image on the screen of my tumor, one thought came to mind … VAMPIRE.

Perhaps it was all the vampire books and movies I've watched in the past jumping to the forefront of my mind as I traced the large, sharp edges on the top and bottom right of the picture screen, yet the only thing I could think of was that I had a large vampire tumor inside of me, and his name was Vladimir.

I don't know if other patients name their tumors, though according to my doctors they've yet to have a patient that's done so; however, I saw Vladimir as a very important aspect of my life — one that would be with me for as long as I lived. It felt only natural to name it. And Dracula's name — Vladimir — was the only name that fit.

In hindsight, it was a prophetic name as I had so much blood drawn for one test or another in the first five months following my diagnosis that I could probably start my own small blood bank.

On a side note, I recently learned that Vladimir means "a great peacemaker" in Russian. Ironically, despite all the chaos in my life caused by Vladimir, in a strange peculiar way he's also brought me a sense of peace. (More on that later.)

Just eight days after seeing the doctor — February ninth — I had a biopsy of the lump performed. In retrospect, I have to laugh when I recall the conversation I had with the pathologist that day. She stated that she could tell the cells she extracted were cancerous; however, she couldn't officially tell me I had cancer until she ran the test and received scientific confirmation. She then asked if I wanted to return to the hospital the following day so she could give me the official results and confirm my cancer diagnosis, or if I preferred, she could merely call me on the phone and provide me with the results then.

I opted to save myself the drive in to the hospital and the seemingly endless wait times, and just have her confirm the results she had already given me over the phone.

I didn't realize tears were rolling down my face until the technician assisting her handed me a box of tissues. She tried to offer comfort, telling me I was strong and could get through this. Yet all I could think was, "How do you know I'm strong? You don't even know me!"

She didn't know that all the women in my family diagnosed with cancer had died, nor the fact that I had no one to help me through this ordeal. I had just gotten my business to where it was lucrative, and now I was facing surgery that I couldn't afford and had no one to take over in my absence. This disease could bankrupt me — even worse, kill me.

Be strong?

That wasn't an option.

It was a requirement!

My wish at that moment was to stick my head in the sand for a few days and pretend this wasn't happening to me. Yet, that wasn't possible. In just two days' time, I was scheduled to conduct my Primal Passion Workshops at Caliente Resorts in Florida. Not something I could postpone at that late date nor did I want to. I couldn't think of a better place to relax and contemplate what I would do and start preparing mentally for the terrifying road ahead. Because of my recent biopsy, I couldn't take advantage of the magnificent pools they had to offer; however, I could lie under the Florida sun and try to pretend for a few more days that I wasn't sick.

I discovered that I not only had breast cancer but my genetic tests revealed I also had a rare mutation in my CHEK2 gene which makes me susceptible to several other forms of cancer, including ovarian, colon and thyroid cancers. (If I had been born a man, prostate cancer would be on the agenda as well.)

As the weeks went by, I became obsessed with learning everything I could about breast cancer and genetic testing, as well as ovarian, colon and thyroid cancers.

I struggled with my fears and my determination to persevere. I had to — I was totally alone. My son literally lived across the world from me. He was in Seattle, Washington, and I was in New York City. He had just moved to the West Coast four months earlier to start his new life and career with his girlfriend. I was estranged from my family and my friends; all lived in different states.

Because I traveled extensively for work, conducting workshops and speaking engagements throughout the U.S. and Latin America, and had spent 16 to 18 hours a day for the past four years building my company, my local friendships had suffered, and most of the people I knew were work related and not someone I could call for a shoulder to cry on.

A few short weeks after my diagnosis and my trip to Florida, I was off to appear at a conference in Seattle; best of all, I was hosting my company's first West Coast conference—something I couldn't cancel and didn't want to.

While in Seattle, I took the opportunity to see my son for my birthday and share the news with him in person. "I have cancer," was not something I wanted to tell him over the phone.

Regrettably, I was a bit "crazed" the first few weeks after my diagnosis — so crazed Bridezilla would have run away in tears if she had to spend time with me.

I was happy one moment and crying the next. I burst into tears at the beauty salon when the woman was washing my hair because I thought to myself, "This could be the last time I ever get my hair washed and colored."

Tears rolled down my face as I stared out the plane window thinking, "What if I never take another trip again?"

When I held my son in my arms, I was very proud of the fact that I held it all together so we could enjoy a few days together before I revealed the news.

When I did reveal the news to my son, he merely nodded his head and walked out of the hotel room to smoke a cigarette. When he returned, he was withdrawn and didn't speak to me for a few days. With much embarrassment, I will admit, I drove my son nuts. In my fear, I lashed out at him and for that I'll be eternally sorry. It's common to take out our fears on those we love because we hope they'll understand and somehow, help make the situation better. Yet, it's still not appropriate, especially given the fact that they have their own fears to contend with.

My son took my craziness in stride. He never argued with me; just remained quiet riding out the "crazy storm." He wrote me a brief note on my birthday card which told me everything I needed to hear, and my fear dissipated for a little while. Now every time I need a little extra courage, I re-read his words and push forward.

His card read,

"Dear Mom, I know you're going through a lot right now and are scared, and I'm sorry that it seems like I don't care. I'm scared too. You've

always been there for me, and the idea of you not being there anymore is a bit too much for me to wrap my head around."

So now I take his silence for what it is — his fear. Fear of losing me and apprehension at not knowing the right words to share with me.

I much prefer his silence than the platitudes from others. Though people mean well, I prefer they say, "I'm not sure what to say to you at a time like this," or "Gee, Charley, it sucks that you have cancer," instead of what they often say.

"It doesn't matter if they cut off your breasts, you don't need them to live."

That comment is as idiotic and offensive as me saying, "It's OK if they cut off your arm, you still have another one."

Or, "So what if your dog of umpteen years died, you could always go out and buy another one."

How insensitive can people be?

Breasts aren't just breasts for a woman! They're part of who we are, how we think of ourselves, how we relate and are viewed by others. Our breasts are life giving as we use them to nourish our children. They're sensual and passion fulfilling as we enjoy the way our lover touches us or we touch ourselves.

Yes, I know people aren't purposely trying to be mean or inappropriate with their comments; all too often, they merely don't know what to say to us. They don't understand the magnitude of breast cancer and how it attacks a woman's self-esteem or her core identity and the beliefs she holds about herself. How it can make you feel vulnerable and undesirable when your breasts are removed.

Ironically, I was in the process of scheduling a Body Love Retreat in Mexico when I was diagnosed with breast cancer. The Body Love Retreat was a new program I developed to help women gain more comfort with their bodies and enhance their sensual divinity. (Yes, I will be conducting Body Love Retreats in the near future with a few special segments specifically for women with breast cancer.)

I believe God, the Goddess, the Universe and whatever Higher Power is out there wanted me to understand what it's like to have breast cancer to better understand what truly loving yourself, your body and accepting life is all about. Okay, maybe that's getting a little too esoteric. I'll admit, I am a bit hooky and spiritual in my beliefs.

No, I don't see cancer as a gift. Far from it! It's more like a pain in my ass — or I should say, pain in my chest.

My life has taken an entirely different path since my diagnosis. I not only see life from a totally new perspective, I also value it more fully.

I do believe that much like cardiac patients, I contributed in some way to my breast cancer diagnosis. I did this through my bad health habits of poor diet and unhealthy eating patterns, not exercising, partying a little too much, as well as other vices I participated in throughout the past 40 years of my life which may have activated my genetic mutation and caused the breast cancer.

Yet, just because I now have breast cancer, doesn't mean my life is over. It's just beginning — anew!

I've made so many radical and wondrous changes in my life, including the ways I treat and interact with others; what I eat and put into my body; the amount of sleep and exercise I engage in daily; even the stress I allow in my life. I really have become a different person. That old adage, *your body is your temple; treat it with respect,* has never been truer nor more significant in my life.

Sometimes, I see my life now as a new life — a new beginning — the post-cancer me. You'll catch me saying things like,

I used to eat that …

I used to drink that …

I used to do that …

… and now I don't do that anymore.

It's not because I can't do it, eat it, or drink it; it's because I choose not to!

I believe, if it's not healthy or rewarding to my life and my health, it doesn't belong.

Choose for yourself what you'll bring into your new life (both current and post-cancer). How will you choose to live?

As I've walked along the path of breast cancer, I've experienced many facets of life and of the world around me. To call this journey "The Insanity of Cancer" would be an understatement. There are many facets to this journey and though I (and you) have no choice but to accept some of them, I've rebelled fervently against others.

Breast Cancer: From Diagnosis to Surgery and my Cancer Tamer Television Talk Show series (available to view on our website and YouTube) are a direct result of the anger and frustration I've experienced at the incredulous views of physicians and health-care providers who claim to want to help, yet expect us to follow blindly. I've experienced for myself, as well as heard many horror stories, of physicians using guilt or shame to keep you towing the line and following their treatment plan. Others dismiss you completely or refuse to treat you, stubbornly sitting before you with their arms crossed and refusing to speak because you hurt their feelings — or ego, — and you had the audacity to ask questions; as one radiologist did to me. (But that's a story for later.)

Shortly after my cancer diagnosis, I was referred to an endocrinologist (thyroid specialist) as a sonogram evaluation discovered the presence of several nodules (lumps) on my right thyroid. That physician sat before me and stated he was going to wait, "until it turned into full blown cancer before taking action."

WTF?

I was sure I must have misunderstood him. Perhaps there was a language barrier since it was clear English wasn't his first language. When I asked him to explain what he'd said, he stated, "Nobody dies from thyroid cancer. We're going to wait to treat it until it's full blown."

Okay, I'll admit, my outburst in response to his comment wasn't the most appropriate.

"Are you stupid?"

I'll concede that yelling that comment at him wasn't the best course of action nor was there any doubt it negatively impacted the next few moments of our interaction. (I'm sure you already deduced that I've never returned to that physician.)

I can't help but wonder, how many other patients he gave that same medical advice to? How many others have walked out of his office unable or too scared to question him or demand a second opinion (as I did); only to return a few months or years later with dire symptoms, or worse yet, incurable cancer?

We've been trained to believe that physicians know best. Hell, they go to school for decades to learn this stuff, right? It makes sense that we should believe in them and defer to their judgement. However, deferring to their judgment after you've taken a little responsibility for yourself and done some research on your condition is better than following blindly.

Burying your heads in the sand is not going to help cure you nor help you create a new life — post-cancer. You must take control and become an active participant in your care. Seek answers and ask questions. Avoidance will only get you so far and make you feel helpless and vulnerable and lead to lack of motivation and depression. Thus, take back control and discover your inner strength.

I recall being told at one point to STOP doing research into breast cancer and the surgeries planned by a nurse navigator because she felt I was asking too many questions. I was so offended — royally pissed off — at such a request. The audacity of her comment still astonishes me. She was supposed to be an advocate for me and assist me through this insanity, and yet, she wanted to shut me down.

It's as if the medical professionals would rather we meekly go about being chopped up (have our breast and ovaries removed), undergo whatever treatment they prescribe and agree with them without raising a fuss or asking questions even when we know something is wrong with our bodies or our proposed care.

Some physicians will take offense and feel we're questioning their education and knowledge; like the pathologist that reviewed the second ultrasound I had performed because the tumor seemed larger just two months after the biopsy. He and his accompanying technician spouted their years of experience after I questioned their results that there had been no change in tumor size. I could only reply with, "you may have 20 years' experience reviewing tumors, but I've had 50 days' experience looking at and feeling only my tumor, and based on a comparison of both these screens, it appears my tumor has grown." (Yes, it was later determined that my tumor had grown two centimeters after the biopsy due to edema and the aggressiveness of my cancer.)

In the months following my diagnosis, I have not only been a patient, I have been an observer as well. I've seen so many women — breast cancer patients — appear beaten down by their medical condition and complications. Cancer tends to erode your self-esteem and zest for life. That very fact, along with the complacency required by some medical providers, has motivated me to rebel against the drone mentality and requirement. This was the very reason the Cancer Tamer Television Talk Show, as well as this Breast Cancer Book Series, were created: to educate, empower and inspire cancer patients.

Please know, I am not stating all physicians are horrible or complacent or tyrants; some are; however, there are others who are compassionate and encourage your involvement. I've had several of these involved in my health care and as guests on my show.

Never forget you have the right to pose questions and request answers, second opinions, and to do your own research. Your life may depend on it.

You have the right to accept or deny treatment options and request a second — even third — opinion or seek alternatives which adhere to your lifestyle and spiritual beliefs.

You have the right to be treated with respect and dignity! Never forget, you are a human being first and a cancer patient second.

Don't sit idly by and allow another to run your life or determine the quality with which you will live it. Yes, cancer is scary, even terrifying at times. Yet, only you can decide the type of patient you will be.

Will you follow meekly along and let others tell you what the best options are for you? Or will you research and ask questions and fight for what you need — or enlist the assistance from family and friends to fight for you when you're a little exhausted by it all? Either choice is fine. It's your choice! Be conscious of it and know that you can fluctuate between your options at any time.

If you take nothing else from this book, know that CHOICE is the key to your recovery.

Breast Cancer: From Diagnosis to Surgery is not about providing you with medical advice. I'm not a medical physician. My doctorate is in human sexuality and psychology. My purpose in writing this book is to share with you what worked for me and hopefully help you avoid some of the pitfalls I experienced. This book is my way of helping you navigate through the insanity called cancer.

Breast Cancer: From Diagnosis to Surgery will provide you with valuable information on what you can expect; questions to ask your physicians and issues you'll need to consider, both emotional and legal. You'll have pages to jot down important information which you'll need to share when interacting with physicians, social workers and your insurance company.

In addition, I will share numerous tidbits of information and ideas which I found helpful during my own breast cancer experience. Though this book and the entire Breast Cancer Book Series is geared toward women diagnosed with breast cancer, it can be used for other types of cancers as well.

This is not a book about treatment options, nor is it intended to provide medical advice. *Breast Cancer: From Diagnosis to Surgery* and the entire series is about what you can do, what will happen, and how to persevere to live a fulfilling life and find your own peace, as well as tame your cancer despite the numerous challenges which come your way.

I've separated the vast information you'll need to navigate your cancer journey into three specific aspects of the cancer journey you are about to embark upon. You'll discover many of the benefits and pitfalls that may occur along the way. Don't worry, you won't be alone.

In essence, we are taking this journey together as each book is written after I've completed each phase of my own journey. Here are the names of each book in the series:

Breast Cancer: From Diagnosis to Surgery
Breast Cancer: From Surgery thru Treatment (coming 2018)
Breast Cancer: Recovery and Beyond (coming 2019)

For now, at the beginning of your cancer journey, I want to impart another piece of advice that I discovered the hard way. Be sure to provide yourself with a much-needed emotional break whenever possible. Don't wait until you feel you "really" need it or "have time for it." Pencil a Mental Health Wellness Day into your calendar weekly. On second thought, write it in with a permanent marker! Even if it's only for an hour or 15 minutes, as a minimum.

This mental health time will be especially helpful during the beginning — once you've been newly diagnosed — and feel like an expiration date has been stamped onto your lifeline.

It's also helpful when you're recovering from surgery and feel like you're not doing enough, nor healing fast enough. (Keep in mind, the more you rest and relax, the faster you'll heal.)

Breast Cancer: From Diagnosis to Surgery was deliberately created to fit easily in your purse or back pocket so that you may carry it with you to appointments and have all your important information at your fingertips.

I encourage you to purchase two large loose-leaf binders. In one, place copies of all your medical notes, test results, even blood work. If you've received more than one cancer diagnoses, you can divide it up with tabs. In the second binder, place copies of your insurance correspondence, bills and other information. There should also be a section on social service organizations and resources such as Social Security Disability Insurance, human resources and the Department of Veterans Affairs (VA) — for vets. You'll be amazed at how quickly these binders fill up.

You'll also want to purchase a journal book or composition notebook to document all your doctors' appointments, the reason for the visit and a brief synopsis of the results. Don't forget to date each entry and include the physician's name or tests you underwent. Personally, I was on my second composition notebook within five months. These notebooks will be a great source of reference for you as time goes by. And though you may pride yourself on your fabulous memory and attention to detail, the magnitude of what you are experiencing — and will continue to experience in the months or years ahead — will jumble your recollection skills, even make you feel a little crazy at times. These notebooks and binders will alleviate a lot of stress as well and provide a record for your loved ones of what's going on in your care.

I invite you to email me and share your thoughts and comments on ways to improve the information in this series and share any tidbits you've discovered along the way.

One final word of advice before you move onto the rest of the book. I know from experience being a lone wolf in this arena is not healthy. Thus, I highly recommend you join a cancer support group in your area or online which resonates with you. Several of the women you'll meet in the support group will become valued friends and a source of education and inspiration for you. Though each of us undergoes her own journey, you are not alone.

Being diagnosed with cancer can be hell, but your life doesn't have to be! This is your opportunity to start anew. Make this second half of your life's journey what you want it to be! Choose for yourself how you will live it.

Live with **ROARING** passion,

Doctor Charley ...

CHAPTER 1

Discovery & Diagnosis

I had to wait 43 days after discovering the lump in my right breast before I could see a physician. My new medical insurance didn't kick in until then. I would have had to wait another two to three weeks before I could be scheduled for a mammogram and ultrasound. Luckily for me, I had called ahead and assured the breast imaging center I would have the required referral documentation, with all the appropriate language.

My mammogram and ultrasound both revealed there was a large mass measuring over 3.9 centimeters in my right breast, and they immediately required a biopsy of it.

On February 9, 2016, the pathologist conducted the biopsy. She thought I was in pain because I kept moving every time she raised the machine and injected the needle into the site to obtain the required biopsy sample. I explained to her that I wasn't in pain, I just wanted to see Vladimir and what the procedure was doing to him. To which she replied, "Charley, it's more important that I see what I'm doing as I perform the biopsy." Okay, I had to give her that one. We both laughed, and she continued the procedure without further movements from me.

Yes, many aspects of this process can and will be frightening. However, it's up to you how you process them emotionally and psychologically. If you don't like your emotions, change them. That's right, simply refocus your thoughts and make a conscious choice about the emotional impact you wish to feel, then strive to maintain that focus.

Personally, I chose humor over vulnerability and feeling helpless. Humor is one of my coping skills. Once I was diagnosed with cancer, and I saw how "serious" everyone else was around me, I took (and still take) great joy in teasing and joking about my disease. That's not to say that I haven't had my meltdowns; I have. However, I've learned to find joy in simple things.

The first day I met my plastic surgeon during the initial phase of my diagnosis was one of the funniest. As this thirty-something-year-old male plastic surgeon sat in a chair before me, examining my breasts and deciding which surgical procedure would work best for me, I asked him what type of sensations I could expect to have in my breasts after surgery. He informed me that the sensation would return to my left breast (the non-cancerous one); however, my right breast would probably never have any sensation whatsoever due to the extent of the area that needed to be excised. I stared at him for a moment, shocked by his reply, then said the first thing that came to mind. "Then you'd better feel me up now so I remember what it's like."

He dropped my breasts and pushed his chair back so fast it banged into the back wall. I burst into laughter as did the nurse in the room with us. Yeah, it's times like these that will help keep you going in the difficult months ahead.

You need to find out for yourself what your best coping mechanism is. Whether it's laugher, journaling, talking with friends or a host of other positive ways to function, then do it often. Anger, tears and feeling sorry for yourself will only get you so far and aren't very constructive. Plus, they lead to stress

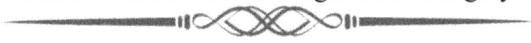

and emotional pain. Therefore, choose a positive form of coping. If you're not sure what that is, explore or seek out a counselor to help you discover a few ways that will work best for you.

Below, jot down three to five positive ways you can cope with stress or innovative new ways you'd like to try. It's useful to have more than one. You'll discover that one way works best during certain situations and another is better during other times. There's no right or wrong way.

If you're struggling or merely need someone to speak to, your physician can refer you to a therapist, social worker or support group. The American Cancer Society hosts a 24/7 hotline where you can speak to one of their trained volunteers, and the VA has a veterans hotline that's also available 24/7 (www.veteranscrisisline.net). Just because you turn to another for help or a shoulder to cry on doesn't make you weak. In fact, it makes you stronger as you receive the emotional support you need to continue and overcome the next hurdle.

_____

_____

_____

_____

_____

As you begin your breast cancer journey, you'll undergo a plethora of tests and evaluations. After each, take a moment to jot down information about your diagnostic tests and their results. The results of some of the tests will determine the course of some of your medical care and medications prescribed.

You will be asked for this information often. Become familiar with the importance of the results from these examinations and the frequency with which they may need to be repeated in the months and years ahead.

Let's get started

Name Your Tumor (optional)
Feel free to give your tumor a name, if you wish. I did. There's nothing wrong with that. This is your disease. You set the parameters.

_____

Discovery
Who discovered the tumor? (You, your lover, a doctor, a mammogram exam, etc.?)

_____

Date of Discovery

_____

Date of Diagnosis
This is the date your physician stated cancer was diagnosed.

_____

ER/PR/HER2 Neu (Indicate whether positive or negative)
This is discovered through a blood test and is significant in your treatment. You'll be asked this question often.

Estrogen _____

Progesterone _____

HER2 Neu _____

Mammogram
This examination can be a bit painful as the technician will pull and push your breasts in various positions, not to mention how

they "squeeze" them in the machine. Good thing breasts are pliable. If you are in extreme pain, discuss this with the technician. Also, be sure to let them know if you have any implants. (It is your right to refuse this examination if you feel it would be detrimental to your health, or you do not believe in them. We'll discuss this further later.)

Date/Results:

_____
_____
_____
_____

Ultrasound/Sonogram

This test is painless. It's performed with you lying down on a gurney. They lower the lights, and the technician performing the test smears a bit of gooey gel onto your breasts (or other area being examined such as your stomach for ovarian cancer). The gel allows the probe to glide more easily over your breasts and provide the feedback the machine needs. This is where you'll be able to get a good look at your tumor. Of course, you can also see it on the mammogram x-rays as well.

You are entitled to a copy of these results and the pictures or scans. I took a picture of the screen with my smartphone. It's now displayed on my wall. Although, I don't share my cancer diagnosis with everyone, I don't hide it like a dirty little secret either. It just is.

Date/Results:

_____
_____
_____
_____

Genetic Testing

Though Genetic Testing is often erroneously referred to as the *BRCA* Test because the BRCA1 and BRCA2 genes are well known for their association with breast cancer, these are merely two of the 24 genes they test for which are associated with various forms of cancer. (This is the same test used for men as they can also be diagnosed with breast cancer and other forms of this disease.)

If cancer runs in your family, having a genetic test performed can provide you with valuable information on conditions to watch out for. Yes, your insurance company will pay for genetic testing if cancer runs in your family and your physician requests it.

Aside from a check swab and the blood tests, this evaluation is painless. It consists of the genetics counselor conducting an interview and jotting down your family history, and identifying cancer and other chronic illnesses in your family. Once the results of the tests are received, you'll know if any of the 24 genes associated with breast cancer or other forms of cancer were detected. (It's a good idea to take a family member with you for this consultation as they may be able to fill in some of the blanks you don't know or recall.)

Keep in mind that just because:

(a) You may have tested positive for the BRCA1 or BRCA2 gene, but that **does not** mean you will get breast cancer in the future (if you don't already have it). It merely signifies you are at higher risk. The same is true of other genes which may be identified with other cancers.

In a way, knowing you have the gene(s) is beneficial because you now have justification for your insurance company to allow you to be monitored more closely and have tests performed on a regular basis, including tests which they may not normally conduct if you had not tested positive.

(b) If you are diagnosed with any rare mutations — as I was — you can check for specialized research studies being conducted you might be able to join.

If you test positive for any genes, you may also wish to have your loved ones genetically tested and monitor their health. Plus, you now have the justification needed for your insurance company to conduct these tests. (For instance, because of my CHEK2 gene mutation, I must have bi-annual ovarian and thyroid tests performed to monitor for cancer, and my insurance is obligated to perform these tests. Whereas, in other individuals, the screening might be conducted in two to five year intervals, if at all.)

Date/Results:

_____
_____
_____
_____

Breast Biopsy

A breast biopsy is performed by cutting a small incision into your breast(s) in the area of the tumor. Cells are extracted and sent to the laboratory. You should have the "official" results in one to three days. Most facilities conduct the biopsy through guided imagery where a machine injects a needle into your breast(s) and retracts it immediately. The biopsy site will be numbed so you probably won't feel anything other than a little pressure in the area. Speak with the pathologist performing the procedure if you have questions or experience any discomfort. Afterward, you'll need to keep the area clean and avoid baths (not showers), pools or Jacuzzis for a week or two. This is to prevent infection. Ask the pathologist for specifics on your timeframe.

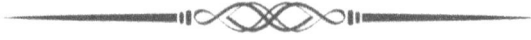

Date/Results:

_____

_____

_____

_____

MRI Tests

This machine is loud. It's so loud they actually provide you with a headset and/or ear plugs to drown out some of the noise. If you're lucky, they'll have good music for you to listen to. If not, hum along to the music anyway. It'll keep you from going bonkers as you lie in that funky biker position for almost an hour while they take the images, add the contrast to your bloodstream and take more pictures of your breasts. (Yes, you're entitled to a copy of these results and any other tests performed. Add them to your loose-leaf binder.)

Date/Results:

_____

_____

_____

_____

PET Scan

This test requires you eat no sugar or carbs for 24 hours prior to your examination as you need to keep your blood sugar count below 300. If it's higher than that, they'll send you home. You'll want to dress with loose, comfortable clothing which has no metal. Thus, avoid jeans, shirts or jackets and wear a pair of sweat pants and a T-shirt instead. If you must wear a bra, use a sports bra with no snaps. Dressing this way will allow you to keep your clothing on as opposed to those hospital gowns that have horrible back drafts. Leave your jewelry at home or take it off prior to the examination, including rings and necklaces.

This test will take x-rays/pictures from your head to your knees. (Not sure why they don't go all the way down your calves and to your toes.) The test begins with the nurse checking your glucose level. If your blood sugar is within acceptable limits, they'll put in your port where they'll inject the medication needed, a little radioactive sugar that'll glow in your PET Scan x-rays. The port is basically a needle placed into you vein which will allow them to put the medicine in later. If your sugar glucose is too high and they can't lower it to an acceptable level, they'll send you home and reschedule you.

After your port is in place, you'll be taken to a "quiet room" where you'll receive the solution and then rest/wait for about 30 minutes. No music, reading nor company is allowed. No need to panic, they merely want you totally relaxed and your blood pressure at optimum. I was put in a Lazy-Boy recliner with a blanket over me and fell asleep — it's a wonderful time for a nap or meditation.

Once you're ready, the nurse will take you into the room and have you lie down on a very narrow table, have you place your arms by your sides and strap you in. Yes, you'll discover what it feels like to be a burrito. (Remember humor is my coping mechanism.)

For the next 30 to 40 minutes, the table you're lying on will move back and forth within this tube. The back and forth motion is gradual and reminiscent of a rocking motion. (It made me fall asleep.) No need to worry about feeling claustrophobic as both ends are open. However, if your nose itches, it'll stay that way until the test is over. Once completed, your physician should have the results in a few days.

Date/Results:

_____

_____

_____

_____

Ovarian Transvaginal Sonogram

This examination consists of inserting a long probe inside your vagina. Typically, the technician will lubricate the six to eight-inch probe and ask you to insert it yourself while you lie back on the examination table. Like the sonogram, images will be taken of your ovaries and uterus to detect any lumps or tumors. It may also detect abnormalities in the lining of the uterus.

Aside from being a little humiliating, this examination should not cause any discomfort. This test should be performed every six months to a year if you have any abnormal findings or if your genetic test results are positive for high risk/susceptibility to ovarian cancer or low malignant ovarian cancer.

Ovarian cancer is often diagnosed in its late stages and leads to higher risks and dire consequences. Thus, be sure you're tested annually!

Date/Results:

_____

_____

_____

_____

Endometrial Biopsy

This examination can be a bit painful. A sample of your uterine wall lining is needed to determine if there are cancer cells present. Though this biopsy is very similar to having a pap smear, and a speculum is inserted into your vagina, the physician goes one step further — going inside the uterus to obtain the necessary cell samples. Your gynecologist will prescribe a pill to help your uterus dilate which you'll take the night before the examination. You may experience a little bleeding after the examination. (Nothing that a panty liner won't keep under control.) However, if you experience a heavy blood flow or major cramps, contact your doctor immediately.

Your test results should be back in the next few days/week and you'll discover if you have any issues and/or endometriosis; this is a thickening of the uterine lining which can lead to cancer and may need to be removed. (Older, mature women do have a thicker lining.)

Discuss the necessary options with your physician. Sometimes, as in my case, they may allow the thickened lining to remain as your body may not be able or ready for additional surgery. Only you and your physician can weigh the options, risks and necessities based on your individual circumstances. Always ask questions and for clarification even, if that means getting a second or third opinion and further testing.

This procedure had me going to the mall for some major retail therapy. I highly recommend you treat yourself afterwards and do some fun and loving self-care!

Date/Results:

_____
_____
_____
_____

Colonoscopy

This examination begins with you drinking a huge jug of medicated water — yep, the whole jug! The mixture (medicine) is already inside the jug, you merely add the water. I'll warn you now, it tastes horrible, yet you must drink it all to ensure an accurate evaluation.

Basically, this mixture is a super strong laxative formulated to flush your colon and get it as clean as possible prior to your examination the following day. The upside is there's no painful cramping.

When they caution you to be close to the bathroom once you begin drinking from the jug, they're not exaggerating. You will be running to the bathroom repeatedly, even minutes — if

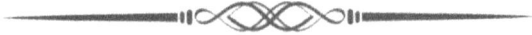

not seconds — after you've just gone. Drinking this funky water completely will allow the doctor (gastroenterologist) to see inside your colon clearly and discover any polyps, tumors or diverticulitis you may have.

The bad news is that no matter how many times you rush to the toilet, you will not lose 20 or 30 pounds like those old TV/radio commercials declared. There really are not 20 to 30 pounds of undigested food or red meat in your colon. You will lose approximately three or four pounds, but nothing to run out and get a new wardrobe over.

You'll be asleep throughout the procedure and your physician will typically give you a rundown of how things went after you're awake. However, the official findings for any polyps removed may take a few days. You will need someone to drive you home as you'll be a little loopy from the anesthesia.

Date/Results:

_____
_____
_____
_____

Thyroid Cancer Screening

Screening for thyroid cancer starts with a sonogram. This is painless, and like the ultrasound previously mentioned, the technician will spread a little gel on your throat, run a probe over your throat/thyroid and take pictures. If there are any nodules detected, they'll know immediately. If nodules (lumps) are detected, you'll be sent to the pathologist for a fine needle biopsy.

The fine needle biopsy is quick and relatively painless, although you will feel slight discomfort and pressure in your throat. I'm talking quick like in 60 seconds or less.

I'll caution you not to look at the needle as that might be a little nerve-wracking. The examination itself is quite simple.

The pathologist inserts a needle into your thyroid and removes a few cells.

The pathologist will be able to tell you immediately if there's a problem and if a more in-depth analysis needs to be performed. Typically, this evaluation is performed once every year or two, more often if necessary or you're being monitored for thyroid cancer. Your physician will discuss with you if you need to be monitored more closely.

Date/Results:

_____

_____

_____

_____

Prostate Examination

Although I'm not a man, and this book is written from the perspective of breast cancer in a woman, I wanted to add a little information for men who may also use this book and find it helpful. Like women, men should have a genetic test conducted. Yes, men can suffer from breast cancer, and some of the genes in the genetic testing line-up, such as the *CHEK2* gene, are associated with breast, as well as prostate cancer. (The CHEK2 gene is a rare mutation which I was diagnosed with and the reason why I wanted my son genetically tested as well.)

The prostate examine includes both a blood test to determine the Prostate Specific Antigen (PSA) which is a substance made by your body. The man would also undergo a digital rectal examination. Yep, this is where the doctor inserts a gloved lubricated finger into your rectum to estimate the size of your prostate and feel for any lumps or abnormalities. If there are any concerns with either of these tests, a needle biopsy may be requested.

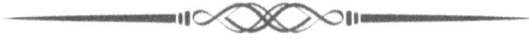

Date/Results:

_____

_____

_____

_____

Bone Density

This evaluation is fairly simple and involves neither pain nor discomfort. Yoga/sweat pants and a T-shirt work best; this way you can keep your clothing on — so long as you do not have any metal on them. And of course, any piercing you may have needs to be removed, though you can check with the technician on what's acceptable.

As you lay on the examination table, a large x-ray machine passes over you. The test takes about 10 to 15 minutes or so. It's amazing to see your skeletal picture.

Note: You will want to establish a baseline on your bone density immediately as the aromatase inhibitors and tamoxifen medications prescribed to block estrogen receptors in your body, as well as other medications, **will** leech calcium from your bones, causing osteoporosis; this is where your bones become brittle and break easily. You'll want to have a bone density test performed every one or two years as osteoporosis will greatly impact your quality of life. (Keep in mind that a bone scan is different than a bone density test.)

Date/Results:

_____

_____

_____

_____

Diabetes Screening

I'm not sure if this is a standard test performed by your physician once you've been diagnosed or not; however, it's one

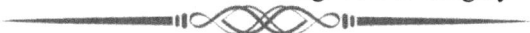

you should discuss with them — especially if diabetes runs in your family — and ensure you're screened for it. Diabetes will greatly impact your surgical recovery and possibly make it more difficult for you to heal. If you are diabetic, it is time to take **complete control** of your eating and exercise habits. It's no longer a matter of convenience or whether or not it's difficult to eat healthy or exercise. This is a matter of life and death, and more so, of whether or not you heal from surgery or suffer major complications.

Date/Results:

_____

_____

_____

_____

Oncotype DX Test

This evaluation is performed **after** your tumor has been removed — not during biopsy. This is where "staging" is assessed. For example, this is where you discover if you are Stage I, Stage II, Stage III or Stage IV. They will also assign a letter to your stage of cancer: "A" if your cancer did not metastasize (spread) into your lymph nodes and "B" if it did. However, if your tumor is very large, they may conduct a more extensive biopsy to obtain these test results immediately. For this test, a sample of your tumor is sent to a special lab, and the results are typically received approximately three weeks after your surgery.

Date/Results:

_____

_____

_____

_____

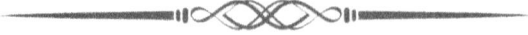

Sweet's Syndrome

Sweet's syndrome is a rare auto-immune disorder which prevents your body from healing after surgery because your white blood cells are on hyperdrive. It is caused from having trauma to an area — such as breast surgery. Sweet's syndrome can cause major complications and even precipitate additional surgery which will only result in further complications.

I was diagnosed with Sweet's syndrome following my second surgery. It wasn't until my plastic surgeon's colleague got involved that I was referred to a dermatologist for evaluation. All my surgeon had to say when he was informed of the diagnosis after returning from vacation was, "After all my years in surgery, I learned something new."

Though I do consider myself "special," there's no way in hell I was the first patient to have suffered from this auto-immune disorder in all his years of practice. I was merely the first one who refused to continue to accept the placating response of "that's normal" during my weekly visits when my skin was rotting away before my eyes, and he refused to act.

Thus, I strongly suggest that if you are not healing after two weeks — three weeks max — following your surgery, or your sutures begin dehiscing (letting go), request an emergency appointment with a dermatologist. This isn't a medical opinion I'm providing, it's one cancer patient's recommendation to another based on personal experience.

Visit our website for more information on Sweet's syndrome: http://cancertamer.org/list-of-shows/sweet-syndrome

Date/Results:

_____

_____

_____

_____

Bi-Annual/Yearly Examinations

List the dates and times of the examinations you need to keep track of throughout the months ahead. Once you've been diagnosed with cancer, yearly or more frequent tests may be required. List those below and keep track of the results. I've listed a few to get you started.

Bone Density

You want to ensure this test is performed every year — or at the very least, no more than two years apart. **Fight for it if you must!** If you are on any type of estrogen blockers (aromatase inhibitors or tamoxifen), these medications literally leech the calcium from your bones, making them brittle and easily broken. It is not a matter of *if* you will get osteoporosis but *when!* Therefore, this test may become a major factor in deciding if it is beneficial for you to stay on certain medications, or determine if they are doing more harm than good.

Date/Results:

_____
_____
_____
_____

Mammograms

Typically, after your surgery (lumpectomy/mastectomy), your breast surgeon will refer you for another mammogram and ultrasound within six months, then once yearly. As a breast cancer patient, you will want to ensure you receive a mammogram and sonogram yearly.

If there were any complications during your surgery, or the need for multiple surgeries, and you're not fully recovered, or able to undergo a mammogram examination because of the breast compression required, speak to your physician about

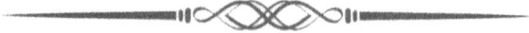

possible alternatives like an MRI or sonogram to ensure there is no recurrence.

Date/Results:

_____

_____

_____

_____

Ultrasound/Sonogram

If you are not completely healed from your surgery or are not comfortable having a mammogram performed, you can opt to have only the sonogram performed. I choose this procedure 10 months after my surgery as I was still recovering on the inside of my chest due to multiple complications. The staff may try to force you or guilt you into getting the mammogram done as well; however, it's up to you to safeguard your health whenever you can. If you do not feel you've healed sufficiently, discuss it with your physician. The ultrasound/sonogram will reveal if there are any issues, and you can then decide if the risks of a mammogram as you continue to heal are warranted.

Date/Results:

_____

_____

_____

_____

_____

OB-GYN Evaluation

Keep an eye out for any abnormal evals and low malignant ovarian cancer. Endometriosis is also a risk for mature women. If you've had issues, a six month eval may be prudent. If not, your yearly check-up should be followed.

Date/Results:

_____

_____

_____

_____

Colonoscopy

These are typically performed every two to three years. If you've had issues, discuss having one yearly with your physician.

Date/Results:

_____

_____

_____

_____

Thyroid Screening

If you are being watched for possible thyroid cancer, an evaluation every six-months may be prudent. My thyroid cancer was discovered during my six-month evaluation and was deemed to be aggressive since it hadn't been detected in my previous exam. Getting it caught early is essential to avoid further complications.

Unlike most cancer patients who fear their follow-up evaluations, I see them as an opportunity to affirm that I'm on my way to a full recovery. If something is detected, then at least we caught it in the early stages and have more options.

Date/Results:

_____

_____

_____

_____

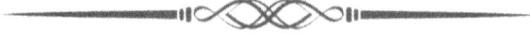

Blood Tests
Date/Results:

_____
_____
_____
_____

Test _____
Date/Results:

_____
_____
_____
_____

Test _____
Date/Results:

_____
_____
_____
_____

Use the following pages to jot down any notes, reminders or comments.

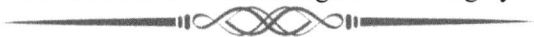

Notes:

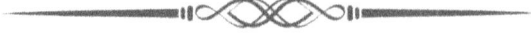

Notes:

CHAPTER 2

Sharing Your Diagnosis

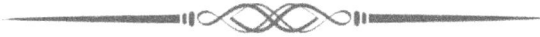

Sharing your diagnosis with others, including your employer or co-workers, is an individual choice. Share that information only when you're ready to do so or when it's absolutely necessary. If your decision is *not to share* your diagnosis with others, that's all right as well. Check in with yourself to ensure not revealing your diagnosis is not because of guilt or shame that you were diagnosed with cancer.

I kept the news of my diagnosis to myself for over two months before I shared it with my son, who was 28 years old at the time. Originally, I had planned not to share the news at all because I didn't want him to worry. He had just moved over 2,800 miles away to start a new career and life with his girlfriend. I didn't feel it was appropriate to ask him to return because I wanted him close by so we could make a few special memories in case something went wrong. (We never stop protecting those we love, right?)

Personally, I believe it's no one's business but those you decide to include in your circle. You can shout it to the world or keep it on a need to know basis. This is entirely your decision. Whatever your choice now, it is perfectly acceptable.

I will warn you that you'll receive a plethora of unsolicited advice once you reveal your cancer diagnosis. You'll hear countless stories about someone's family member or friend who had cancer and how they dealt with it. You'll also be bombarded with a plethora of ailments the person is going through or has experienced in the past — almost as if they are in competition with you, or they're trying to commiserate. In a way, that's very kind of them, yet it might not be what you want to hear at the moment. It's perfectly acceptable to cut them off when necessary.

I don't know about you, but what annoys and exasperates me the most are comments such as, "You're strong; you can fight this." when the person doesn't even know me.

Worse yet are comments from family or friends who adamantly declare, "You don't need breasts. I'd tell them to cut them off me if I had cancer." Yes, I've heard this comment several times from both men and women. And I've wanted to slap them for uttering such a stupid, inappropriate comment.

Take comfort in the fact that they don't mean to be inappropriate; they just don't know what to say, and they're reaching for ways to comfort you. Kindly advise them that they don't need to say anything; or if you're really nice, give them the words you need to hear. This will help reduce your stress in those situations — and theirs.

I will warn you that some family and friends may be overwhelmed by your diagnosis and choose not to interact with you further. That's their loss not yours! They're missing out on an important aspect of your life; one that will change how you see the world and your life, as well as your interactions with others, forever.

Others may choose not to discuss nor acknowledge your cancer diagnosis. For instance, my son doesn't discuss my cancer nor its treatment because of his fear. I understand this, and when we speak on the phone other than telling him I'm doing fine, we talk about other aspects of our lives. I recently learned he was talking to others about my diagnosis. Though it is a little saddening to discover that he'll speak with others but not me, I'm pleased that at least he's building his own source of support and that he cares.

If you have younger children at home, decide the extent of information you will share with them. This is especially important if you're undergoing chemotherapy as they will notice if Mommy loses her hair.

On the other hand, you may have loved ones that become a bit intrusive in their support, demanding to know and see everything, including your sutures and scars during the healing process. They may even make you feel guilty if you don't wish to share. With these individuals, you'll need to establish boundaries, and yes, constantly reinforce them. When exasperated with them, remind yourself they care and mean well.

One benefit to sharing your diagnosis with family and friends is having them assist you in doing research into your condition and treatment options. There's so much to learn and so many intricate facets to cancer that it can be overwhelming to try and cover it all, especially when you're first diagnosed — even months after. Trust me, I've tried.

If you're diagnosed with more than one type of cancer at once, it can become a nightmare (i.e., breast cancer, thyroid cancer, leukemia, etc.).

Let your family and friends help you conduct research. Assign them tasks they can perform. This will provide them with a sense of satisfaction, and yes, even a sense of control as they may also be feeling vulnerable and helpless. In some small way, this will make them (and you) feel safe and a bit more in control of your life. We'll discuss this further in the chapter on *Cancer Tamer Posse.*

Use the space below to jot down the names and contact information of family and friends you'd like to share your diagnosis with. I've also provided a few pages where you can

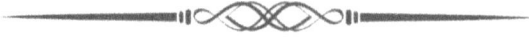

jot down special notes or comments:

Name: _____ Number: _____

Name: _____ Number: _____

Name: _____ Number: _____

Name: _____ Number: _____

Name: _____ Number: _____

Name: _____ Number: _____

Name: _____ Number: _____

Name: _____ Number: _____

Name: _____ Number: _____

Use the following pages to jot down a few additional notes or comments.

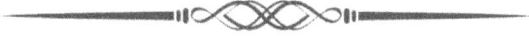

Notes:

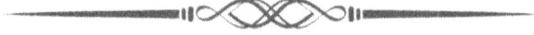

Notes:

CHAPTER 3

Personal Information

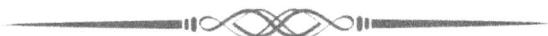

───────────⊰❈⊱───────────

Though you know your personal information, it'll help those assisting you through this journey to have the particulars easily accessible. You can photocopy this information and hand it to the various providers who request it. Everyone will want to know it.

Don't be surprised if you become annoyed with the number of times you'll have to repeat yourself. I've gotten to where I just hand them a synopsis of my condition along with a list of my medications.

You may find it more convenient to simply hand them this book, opened to the appropriate pages, and allow them to review the information for themselves.

Let's Start with the Basics

Below is information you will need to keep handy and up-to-date for physicians and your insurance company. Add any additional information you consider necessary at the back of this section. We'll add medications in the following chapter. I also keep this information on my smart phone under my name.

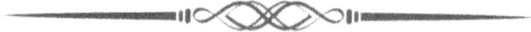

Keep in mind, this information will change sporadically. When you are first evaluated and diagnosed, you'll have countless doctor's appointments and examinations you'll undergo. Keep a separate notebook where you jot down the dates of each appointment and what occurred, as well as the results of any tests performed. I went through two composition notebooks by my fifth month.

For your convenience, I've included blank pages in the back of this book where you can keep notes. Trust me, no matter how great you are at recalling information, there will be times when you can't remember your own name ... smiles.

Your Name:

_____

Your Phone Number:

_____

Insurance Policy Number:

_____

Insurance Telephone Number:

_____

Secondary Policy Number:

_____

Primary Physician:

_____

Nurse Navigator:

_____

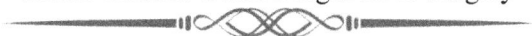
Pharmacy:

_____

Durable Medical Equipment Source: (These are supplies such as heart rate monitors, gauze pads, Xeroform, etc.)

_____

_____

_____

Emergency Contact/Relationship to You:

_____

_____

_____

Health Care Proxy:

_____

_____

_____

Allergies: (List all allergies you have including allergies to various medicines and foods, as well as your reaction to them. (For example: I'm allergic to Benadryl; it gives me seizures; adhesives — including surgical glue. They cause infections and make my skin rot, and blueberries make my lips swell.))

_____

_____

_____

_____

_____

_____

_____

_____

_____

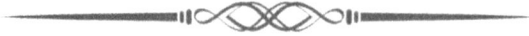

Medical Transportation Number:

_____

_____

_____

_____

Access-A-Ride:

_____

_____

_____

Social Worker/Therapist:

_____

_____

_____

_____

Breast Surgeon:

_____

_____

_____

_____

Second Opinion Breast Surgeon:

_____

_____

_____

_____

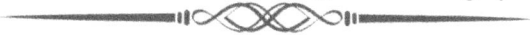

Plastic Surgeon:

_____
_____
_____
_____

Second Opinion Plastic Surgeon:

_____
_____
_____
_____

Oncologist: (You can and should obtain a second opinion for all treatment options, especially when you're looking at chemo and radiation therapies.)

_____
_____
_____
_____

Radiologist:

_____
_____
_____
_____

Dermatologist/Immune Disorder Specialist:

_____
_____
_____
_____

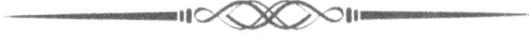

OB/GYN:

_____
_____
_____
_____

Endocrinologist:

_____
_____
_____
_____

Other Specialists:

_____
_____
_____
_____

Use the following pages to jot down any additional physicians and services.

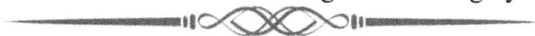

Notes:

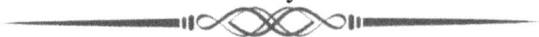

Notes:

CHAPTER 4

Legal Paperwork

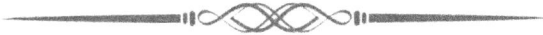

—————⊷⧓⊶—————

Most individuals do not wish to discuss nor consider the possibility of death from a cancer diagnosis nor its complications. Family and friends will reassure you that you'll be fine and even chastise you for bringing up the topic. You may even be apprehensive to broach the topic yourself for fear of upsetting your loved ones or being considered fatalistic.

Unfortunately, death is a very real and valid concern. As an adult cancer patient, it's also one you must be willing to address. Not only that, you need to prepare yourself and those you love for the possible consequences and/or complications of surgery or treatment which may leave you debilitated for a brief time or worst-case scenario — permanently.

To begin with, speak with your friends or loved ones about the need for a health care proxy. This individual will be responsible for ensuring your medical treatment request(s) are followed in the event you are unable to advocate for yourself. This includes situations where you're incapacitated or mentally unable to do so. For example, following your surgery when

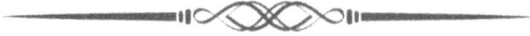

you're groggy and in pain. This individual must be at least 18 years of age.

I would advise against choosing someone as your health care proxy without discussing it with them first. The whole point of having a health care proxy is that this person will carry out your wishes. (You can choose an alternate in case that individual is not available.) Once you've designated the individual, discuss various scenarios and what you wish done.

If complications arise during surgery, the physicians may need to speak with your health care proxy about what needs to be done and what they believe you would have wanted. Thus, it's imperative to discuss possibilities with them. For instance, do you wish extreme measures taken?

Your health care proxy should be someone you trust to carry out your wishes. In the event, you do not have family or friends you wish to designate as your health care proxy, the hospital will assign someone to you. This will not be your physician nor surgeon as that would be viewed as a conflict of interest.

Personally, I chose a friend I trusted as opposed to my son, as I didn't wish to put my son in the position of making a life or death decision where I was concerned. I don't think he'd be able to deal with such a responsibility, or heaven forbid, have to tell the doctors to pull the plug.

Below write in the name, contact information and relationship to you of your health care proxy. Yes, you may designate an alternate or change this individual as needed. Be sure to alert the hospital and you physician's office when making changes.

Health Care Proxy:

_____

_____

_____

_____

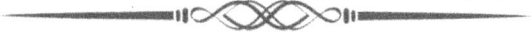

Alternate Health Care Proxy:

_____

_____

_____

_____

A health care proxy is not the only legal aspect you need to consider. You'll also wish to create a living will. A living will, also known as advanced directives is where you state what you wish done if extreme measures need to be taken. For example, do you wish to be placed on life support? If so, is there a time you wish it to end? What if there is no brain activity, but the life support is keeping your heart pumping; do you wish to be taken off life support? Do you wish to donate any viable organs? Do you wish to have a certain type of music played in your room daily if you end up in a coma? Do you wish everything medically possible done before your health care proxy gives the OK to terminate extreme measures?

You will need to contact an attorney to help you create a living will as well as a last will and testament. The difference between the two is that a last will is used when you die, whereas, a living will is used if you become incapacitated and are unable to make medical decisions for yourself.

Warning: You don't want to hide a living will. The living will is there for your benefit. Create a file of important documents and keep it in your nightstand or in your desk drawer.

You can write up a last will and testament on your own or look online and obtain the paperwork for a few dollars, fill in the blanks and then have it notarized. Most banks will notarize a document for free if you are their customer. Some charge a nominal fee. You need witnesses for your last will and testament, therefore check with your bank or other organizations if they will notarize it. There may be a pro bono program for cancer patients in your area that can assist you; check with your state's bar association.

Wills are very important and you want yours to stand up to legal scrutiny; thus, be sure you consult with a legal representative. You can also include a video to play alongside your will. In it, you can provide parting words of wisdom and wishes you'd like for the viewers future, as well as, share your love for them.

Once you have created your last will and testament, place it in a location easily accessible to your loved ones; or in a safe deposit box. You don't want them to have to search for it.

Another alternative, if you don't want anyone reading your will prior to your death, is having your attorney or a trusted friend hold onto it.

Be sure to read your will carefully to ensure your treasures are being passed on to those you love. If you've created a previous will and wish to change the beneficiaries, you must contact an attorney to provide the proper wording necessary to render the old will invalid. Since wills are legal documents, "homemade" ones may not be considered legal or admissible in court — especially if not notarized and witnessed by two individuals who do not profit from it. Thus, contact an attorney to ensure everything is legally binding and your final wishes can be adhered to.

I know hiring an attorney can be expensive and during this time you're probably watching every penny; therefore, contact your hospital social worker, nurse navigator or hospital customer service to determine if they know of any programs available where you can have your last will and testament done for free.

If you're a veteran, check with the VA for possible services and additional programs to help you and your family through the difficult times ahead.

I had my will prepared free of charge by my local councilwoman's office, through a program she sponsored for cancer patients. It was simple and painless. I will admit, I got a bit teary-eyed as I considered the fact that I was signing a paper that would be read when I'm dead. Yet, it made me feel relieved to know that my son and loved ones would have this matter taken care of and no one would need to argue over the dishes and silverware or anything else they wanted.

When getting these services free of charge, you will receive a "basic" will, nothing fancy. That's OK unless you're Donald Trump and have billions of assets — in which case, you'd be able to afford a great attorney. For mine, the attorney wrote up a standard will in which all my belongings went to my beneficiary (my son) and a little money was donated to my favorite charity.

For all my personal property, such as my juke box, records, and book collection, I made a video tape. My video tape also included a few parting words for my loved ones and my hopes and wishes for their future.

On a side note, the Cancer Tamer Foundation provides assistance with filming a video tape to leave a message to your loved ones as mentioned above. We call it *Video of Love & Remembrance.* We're trying to come up with a better name for this service as that name sounds a little fatalistic. Your suggestions are always welcomed. My son suggested we call it "One last thing …" Another possible name to call the video is, "Here and Now." I will admit, Here and Now is my favorite. What's yours? Share it with us at: info@CancerTamer.org

Keep in mind that the video **is not** a legal will. It is merely a way to leave a message to your loved ones and to yourself.

The *Video of Love & Remembrance* is also not your death song. It is a way to remember — to document — what life is like for you at this moment in your cancer journey.

Use the space below to jot down the name of your attorney or the legal representative who created your will. If you've placed a copy of the will in a secure location, safe deposit box or somewhere in your home, state where. If you've

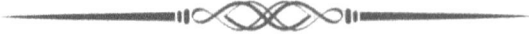

created a video tape, also note that. If you haven't yet made one, write down the name and number of possible avenues you can use to have one created.

Last Will and Testament Attorney or Possible Preparation Services:

_____

_____

_____

_____

Location of Will & Video:

_____

_____

Location of Living Will/Advanced Directives:

_____

_____

Your last will and testament is not the only important paperwork you and your family will need to keep track of during these difficult times. It's a great idea to keep all your important paperwork in one area. I keep all my paperwork such as social security card, will, birth certificate, mortgage deed, even my DD214 (veteran information) and my son's birth certificate in a folder in my work desk. I also keep a folder with all the additional legal papers and financial documents my son will need such as royalty and copyright documentation on my numerous published books, my business documents, credit card and bank information in a special notebook. I will admit there are tons of paperwork I still must gather, however, at least I've started. Just working on one item a day will have you prepared in no time.

Another important document to have is a **power of attorney**. This document provides the person you designate to act on your behalf. They can open bank accounts, manage your finances and act in your best interest. Most powers of attorney have no stipulated end date; however, you can place one. Also, you can revoke the power of attorney at any time. Discuss the legalities and special provisions, if any, with your attorney.

Below I've noted a few of the major items to include/consider putting together in a special folder to make it easier for others (and yourself) to find easily. I recommend purchasing an accordion file if you have lots of documents or using a simple box to keep all your important documents in one location. There's a major sense of relief, control and accomplishment when this is all done.

A List of Significant Items to Include

Location of Legal & Important Paperwork:

_____

_____

Mortgage(s)

If you have a VA mortgage, you may be able to lower your interest rate. It may take a little discussion with the mortgage/insurance provider; however it's so worth it. (Note: this reduction is not a refinancing, merely a reduction in your interest rate which then reduces your mortgage payments. Rare but possible.)

_____

_____

Mortgage Insurance

Check your insurance paperwork as some insurance coverages built into the mortgage will cover you if you're unable to work

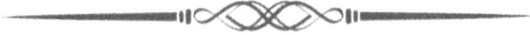

due to illness as long as your name is on the deed. Every little bit helps, right?

_____

_____

_____

Life Insurance Policy: (if more than one, list them all)

_____

_____

_____

_____

Automobile Registration/Car Insurance Information

_____

_____

_____

Safe Deposit Box

_____

_____

_____

Personal Checking/Savings Accounts

_____

_____

_____

Business Checking/Savings Accounts

_____

_____

_____

Credit Cards
Check your credit cards for possible coverage due to health conditions and inability to work. If you paid for this coverage,

contact your credit card company. Typically, all you need to prove your disability is a note from your doctor saying you're unable to work due to health conditions.

If necessary, contact the companies and ask if they'll reduce your payments for a limited time to allow you to keep up with the payments. Many credit cards have a "Hardship Program" which allows reduced payments. They may also work with you to pay a certain amount monthly to bring your account current and enable you to pay it off. Best of all, if you connect with a sympathetic worker, they may reduce or remove the monthly interest charge or late payment charges.

Watch out for additional charges such as adjustment fees which are tacked onto your debt on top of interest charges and late fees.

Some companies will accept a partial settlement payment on your credit card debt; this can range approximately half or less than what you own. However, they may require you to then close the account; which may make it difficult in the future to open a new account. Though at this time in your life you're most likely thinking only of the present and what you need to do in order to keep your head above water and keep the creditors at bay, you don't want to screw up your chances for credit in the future. Check with your accountant or a credit card consulting firm about the impact a settlement payment will have on your credit rating before committing to it.

Inquire about the various options available. Always request to speak to a supervisor if the representative you're speaking with states they can't help you or you feel they are unwilling to help. I always call in the late evening or after midnight as I find the service is better.

Another option is for you to make a settlement payment or make arrangements in a pre-emptive strike to control your debt once you know you're going to start cancer treatment, are going to undergo surgery or if you anticipate complications. Otherwise, wait until it becomes absolutely necessary, as you may need to use your credit cards to cover expenses if you experience treatment complications and are unable to return to work; or if you're self-employed and are unable to perform the work necessary to keep your business afloat and are off work for an extended period of time.

Below jot down the name, number and contact information for each credit card in your name.

_____

_____

_____

_____

_____

_____

_____

_____

_____

_____

_____

_____

_____

_____

Social Security Disability Insurance & Supplemental Security Income

Your doctors cannot really predict how your condition will progress once treatment begins. You can experience complications due to surgery or medication. Once you are diagnosed with cancer, contact the Social Security Administration Disability Office and ask them to provide you with information about the benefits you are entitled to and when you would be able to apply for them. Sometimes, you can begin the paperwork in anticipation of medical necessity. You can also apply online here: www.ssa.gov/disabilityssi/

Foolishly, I thought my cancer treatment would be completed in two to three months. In my mind, I envisioned it like this: two weeks off following surgery and then I'd be

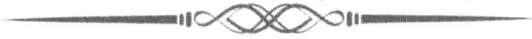

cured. I didn't anticipate the numerous complications I would experience nor the additional surgeries I would require. I also did not anticipate that it would take me over 10 months to recover from complications of my initial surgery, only to be diagnosed with thyroid cancer less than a year later which will require additional surgery.

Even as I write this first book in the Breast Cancer Book Series, I'm not fully recovered from my second surgery and have yet to begin the recommended seven weeks of daily radiation treatments. (I opted not to undergo chemotherapy.)

If you are not employed and are a housewife, you may still be entitled to Supplemental Security Insurance (SSI) or Social Security Disability Insurance (SSDI) through your spouse's plan. (SSI and SSDI are two different plans, and you must file for them separately. You will receive benefits commencing from the date you filed; file when you realize you're going to be off work for over a year.)

You never know what turns your life will take during this insane path called cancer. Therefore, like you would do for any storm, prepare, plan and anticipate.

_____

_____

_____

_____

_____

Veteran's Benefits (VA)

If you're a veteran, regardless of how long it's been since you served, check with your local Veterans Affairs office for possible benefits you may be entitled to, as well as, assistance programs they may connect you with.

_____

_____

_____

_____

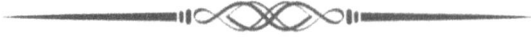

It's never too early to start preparing. Having this information at your fingertips will take a huge weight off your shoulders and provide you with a sense of control and empowerment.

Use the following pages to jot down any additional information and services you feel need to be added to the list.

Notes:

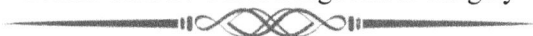
Notes:

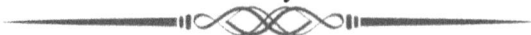

Notes:

CHAPTER 5

Physician Information & Referrals

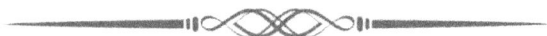

Once you're diagnosed with cancer, life appears to be set on fast-forward and you're merely trying to keep up and not fall off this insane merry-go-round. Don't despair!

The truth is, you'll have plenty of time to obtain the referrals you need and the second and third opinions you may wish to conduct to allow you to be well versed on what's about to happen and what you can expect.

Unless your diagnosis warrants immediate surgery or medical intervention, discuss with your primary physician, surgeon and oncologist options and time constraints. For example, as I work for myself and was conducting two conferences the month after my diagnosis, I couldn't immediately cancel them, nor did I want to. Thus, I had to postpone my surgery for two months.

There are many reasons to postpone surgery, including preparing yourself, your children and loved ones for the necessary care following your surgery and having everything necessary in place. Even more imperative is ensuring you receive the pertinent information and test results necessary for you to make a proper and informed decision.

Do not allow fear to dictate your course of action; you may end up regretting it.

After my diagnosis, I was referred to the breast surgeon. When I arrived for my appointment, I was taken to an examination room and told the doctor would be with me shortly. A few minutes later, a woman in scrubs entered, sat down before me, smiled and said, "So, you're here for a dual mastectomy and ovaries removal."

I looked at her like she had two heads. I shook my head and declared, "You must have the wrong chart."

She looked down at the chart then looked back at me. "You're Charley Ferrer, right?" When I nodded in affirmation, she continued, "Then that's what you're here for."

All I could think to say was, "Who are you?"

That's when she realized she hadn't introduced herself and the nurse with us in the room hadn't performed the introductions either. After a few minutes of discussion where she stated my breast biopsy proved cancerous, I advised her I didn't feel it was appropriate for her to "chop me up" when I merely had one breast that was affected, and they had yet to perform any gynecological tests to determine if my ovaries were cancerous as well. Which, of course, immediately had me thinking I needed to go back to my gynecologist to see what's happening in that arena.

She went on to inform me that as cancer ran in my family, it was best to have a dual mastectomy and ovaries removal; however, if I wished, I could first be tested for the genetic markers, a simple blood test, and meet with the genetics counselor.

I opted to obtain genetic testing to determine if such radical surgery was in fact necessary and requested further tests be performed to determine if other areas of my body were also affected with cancer as the only tests which had been conducted to date were the mammogram and ultrasound — and those tests did not justify such invasive surgical procedures.

I will admit, her comments scared the hell out of me — to think that cancer was not just in my breasts but in other parts of my body as well.

I met with the genetics counselor minutes later as she was available. She took me in to have the required blood and saliva tests, and then we discussed my family's medical history.

Though the genetics test is often erroneously called "the BRCA" test because the two most common genes associated with breast cancer are the BRCA1 and BRCA2 genes, the test actually looks at 24 other genes associated with breast and other cancers. If you're "special" like me, you may have other genes which are mutated and cause a host of other problems, as well as make you more susceptible to other cancers. (Sometimes, it sucks to be special. On the bright side, I am now justified in wearing the X-men's jumpsuit.)

Please keep in mind that just because you have a gene associated with breast or any other type of cancer, it **DOES NOT** mean you will get it. It merely signifies that you are more susceptible and at higher risks to suffer from that particular cancer. However, with preventive care, proper diet and exercise and diligent medical screening, if cancer does pop up its ugly head, you'll be able to detect it sooner and be in better health to deal with it. I highly recommend familiarizing yourself with Dr. Bruce Lipton's work on epigenetics!

By the way, another great benefit to having genetic testing performed is that if you are at higher risk, your insurance will pay for more frequent testing as per recommended protocols for prevention and screening.

The down side to genetic testing is that if you do test positive for other possible cancer genes, you may feel anxious or fearful about contracting an additional cancer. I again refer you to Dr. Lipton's epigenetics teachings and his book, *The*

Biology of Belief, as well as, his videos on YouTube and on his website. www.brucelipton.com.

Always remember that just because you are susceptible to something doesn't mean you'll get it. It's like playing the lotto; just because you buy a ticket doesn't make you a winner.

As for second opinions on surgery, it's imperative to keep in mind that **once you have had surgery, no other surgeon will see you if something goes wrong.** No one wants to step in "someone else's mess."

Thus, ensure to gather all the necessary information now so you are well informed about your options, even if that option is not to have a mastectomy and go with a less invasive procedure like a lumpectomy.

Also speak with your surgeon about their referral protocols should there be any complications.

Regardless of your decision, it's amazing how many physicians and specialists you will be referred to following your cancer diagnosis. Not to mention the various physicians you'll be referred to who specialize in a specific aspect of your cancer or the various medication prescriptions you will receive. This number will double, perhaps triple, if you are diagnosed with more than one type of cancer or experience any complications.

I don't know if you're old enough to remember a time when one physician saw you for all your medical issues. Perhaps, I'm simply dating myself, but I miss those times. On the plus side, having someone who specializes in a separate field will assist you in getting all your concerns addressed as you ask questions, conduct your own research on your condition and move forward with your treatment options.

Many of your physicians will specialize only in one aspect of your care. This is true of your breast surgeon and your plastic surgeon which are two different surgeons. Each will handle a different facet of your surgery.

Don't be afraid to ask questions or to request a second or third opinion — regardless of what insurance company you have. **That's your right as a patient!**

You are also permitted to request a different physician if the one you're assigned does not jive with you. I've requested a new physician on two different occasions, as I did not feel the physicians assigned to my care were appropriate for me. And though some physicians can be worth their weight in gold, others are not.

Pardon me as I use a shoe analogy to illustrate my point. If your shoe didn't fit properly, you'd return it to the store and get another pair, wouldn't you? The same is true with physicians or those handling your treatment and diagnostic testing.

We all know that everyone's personality is unique, and we won't always get along. During this phase of your life, this journey, it's perfectly acceptable to point this out and request someone who does move to the same drumbeat as you — or close to it. With everything else you'll have going on, you don't want to stress every time you go to see "that" doctor.

It's not about hurting someone's feelings when you say, "I'd prefer another nurse or physician." It's about advocating for yourself!

If you feel uncomfortable doing so, ask a friend or loved one to help you. You can always call on the phone after an appointment and request another physician.

I ran into this problem with the radiologist who took over my care while my assigned radiologist (whom I loved) went on maternity leave. He and I clashed instantly. He didn't appreciate it when I had to repeatedly correct him concerning my situation — he never reviewed my chart and thus was not familiar with my special needs due to surgical complications. When I inquired, *"What benefit would I receive from radiation as I am already nine months post-surgery, and it would be another month before I am fully healed?"* he felt I was questioning his expertise and took offense. He then literally sat before me, crossed his arms, and declared, *"I'm not going to talk to you. You've already made up your mind."* Then he proceeded to sit there in silence.

I was flabbergasted!

I tried to smooth over the situation and explained that I wasn't questioning his expertise; I was merely terrified as so many things had already gone wrong with my care, and I didn't want to complicate my condition further. He merely shrugged and continued to stare at me in silence. After another five minutes of complete silence, I told him I was getting dressed and leaving. Yep, I had been sitting there the whole time with my breast hanging out in one of those horrible hospital gowns waiting for him to examine me and provide care.

I shared the situation with the hospital social worker. She was as shocked as I was by his reprehensible behavior. She couldn't believe such a thing happened until I assured her, I had it all on tape if she wanted to listen to it. (I record everything with my iPhone.)

When I requested another physician, I was told there wasn't one and I would need to wait until my primary radiologist returned from maternity leave in approximately two months. I decided to go elsewhere for my treatment.

Yes, if necessary, you can seek care outside the hospital or medical facility you're currently working with. Neither your insurance company nor that physician can prevent you from doing so. All you must verify is that the new facility takes your insurance.

Be sure to have all your paperwork ready for the transfer of your care if that's what you ultimately desire. Then again, you don't need to transfer all your care elsewhere, merely the aspect necessary if there is not another physician who could take over, as was the situation in my case.

On a side note, you should keep a paper copy of all your test results, blood work, surgeries, physician's notes, etc. Create that loose-leaf binder I've repeatedly mentioned. The

American Cancer Society also provides a free Treatment Planner. Contact them for further information on that and other products. These records will be essential if you ever decide to transfer your care to another provider or move residency.

Another important factor that I discovered during my treatment which we'll discuss in greater depth in book two of the series, *Breast Cancer: From Surgery thru Treatment*, is the need for a dermatologist.

Though a dermatologist may not be frequently associated with breast cancer, I found one invaluable during my treatment and recovery. Two weeks following my second surgery which was turning into a nightmarish repeat of the first one, I was referred to a dermatologist by my plastic surgeon's partner (as my plastic surgeon went on vacation after placing surgical glue over my sutures — something I'm highly allergic to). As I previously warned you, surgeons will not see you if you're having complications with someone else's surgery. No one wants to step into anyone else's mess. However, as his colleague, she agreed to see me. I appreciated her honesty when she stated, after the assessment of my condition, that she wasn't sure what was going on and why I wasn't healing. She decided to "look outside the box" of standard post-op care and referred me to a dermatologist to evaluate me for a possible immune disorder or skin condition as the connective tissue disorder biopsy conducted during the second surgery came back inconclusive.

The dermatologist diagnosed Sweet's syndrome.

Yes, "sweet" like in candy.

My initial reaction to that diagnosis was, "Are you kidding me?" (Well okay, I used a few more colorful adjectives.) Not only was I diagnosed with a rare genetic mutation, now I had a ridiculously named immune disorder — Sweet's syndrome.

From my experience and the way my breasts appeared, I would have called it something like, "flesh-eating bacteria," or "Frankenstein's Bride" or "makes holes in chest" syndrome.

Despite its funky comical name, Sweet's syndrome is an auto-immune disorder caused by having extreme trauma to an area. Your immune system kicks into hyper-drive to combat the injury. Because of this hyper-drive effect, your immune system sees everything as the enemy, including healing tissue.

The great news is the dermatologist can provide you with medication to calm down this disorder and begin to normalize your immune system so you can begin healing. Thus, if you experience complications following surgery and you're not healing after two — three weeks max — discuss this option with your physician and request an emergency appointment. Personally, I would recommend having a dermatologist on board from the beginning — **before surgery!**

One more point before I leave you to jot down information, consider recording your appointments. I recorded every appointment I had from the moment I heard the word cancer. The reason for this is that your brain will shut down because it's overwhelmed, and you're afraid. Having the recording handy will allow you to replay it afterwards so you can note all the questions, answers and comments made which relate to your care. I always let my doctors know I was recording as I did not have anyone to go through the process with me, and it would avoid me calling them 10 to 20 times daily with questions.

Recording also allows you to play it for a loved one who couldn't attend the appointment with you. And though you can certainly take notes, a recording is worth its weight in gold as you can listen to it repeatedly.

As you are discovering, cancer comes with numerous doctor's visits and referrals. For your convenience, use the following pages to jot down physicians' contact information, reasons for the referral and brief summaries of the results.

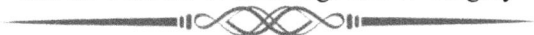

Their contact information will also be helpful when making medical transportation appointments.

Physician's Name: _____

Phone Number: _____

Address: _____

_____

_____

Reason for Appointment:

_____

_____

_____

Date/Time of Appointment:

_____

Comments/Results: _____

_____

_____

_____

_____

_____

Follow-up: _____

Notes:

Dr. Charley Ferrer

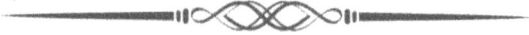

Physician's Name: _____

Phone Number: _____

Address: _____

_____

_____

Reason for Appointment:

_____

_____

_____

Date/Time of Appointment:

_____

Comments/Results: _____

_____

_____

_____

_____

_____

Follow-up: _____

Notes:

Breast Cancer: From Diagnosis to Surgery

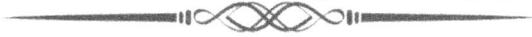

Physician's Name: _____

Phone Number: _____

Address: _____

_____

_____

Reason for Appointment:

_____

_____

_____

Date/Time of Appointment:

_____

Comments/Results: _____

_____

_____

_____

_____

_____

Follow-up: _____

Notes:

Dr. Charley Ferrer

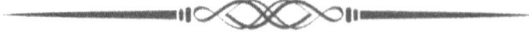

Physician's Name: _____

Phone Number: _____

Address: _____

_____

_____

Reason for Appointment:

_____

_____

_____

Date/Time of Appointment:

_____

Comments/Results: _____

_____

_____

_____

_____

_____

Follow-up: _____

Notes:

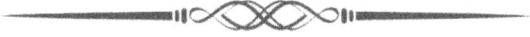

Physician's Name: _____

Phone Number: _____

Address: _____

_____

_____

Reason for Appointment:

_____

_____

_____

Date/Time of Appointment:

_____

Comments/Results: _____

_____

_____

_____

_____

_____

Follow-up: _____

Notes:

Dr. Charley Ferrer

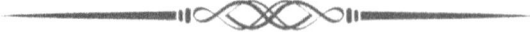

Physician's Name: _____

Phone Number: _____

Address: _____

_____

_____

Reason for Appointment:

_____

_____

_____

Date/Time of Appointment:

_____

Comments/Results: _____

_____

_____

_____

_____

_____

Follow-up: _____

Notes:

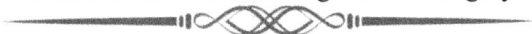

Physician's Name: _____

Phone Number: _____

Address: _____

_____

Reason for Appointment:

_____

_____

_____

Date/Time of Appointment:

_____

Comments/Results: _____

_____

_____

_____

_____

_____

Follow-up: _____

Notes:

Dr. Charley Ferrer

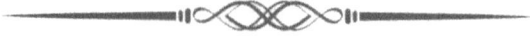

Physician's Name: _____

Phone Number: _____

Address: _____

_____

_____

Reason for Appointment:

_____

_____

_____

Date/Time of Appointment:

_____

Comments/Results: _____

_____

_____

_____

_____

_____

Follow-up: _____

Notes:

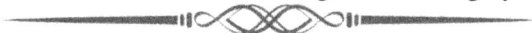
Notes:

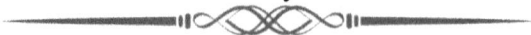

Notes:

CHAPTER 6

Medications & Supplements

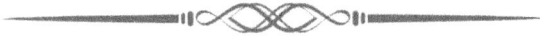

––––––⊪∾⟨✕⟩∾⊪––––––

I t is imperative that you keep track of your medication and any supplements you are taking, including their start/end dates. I keep this information on my smart phone under my emergency information's tab. This way, when I forget or if an emergency occurs, and I'm incapacitated or unable to provide the information myself, it'll still be readily available to first responders and emergency personnel.

Having this information at your fingertips will also come in handy when the physician/clinician you're seeing doesn't know your medical history. This way, you can quickly call it up and let him or his nurse copy it into the chart. (The emergency contact is a feature most smartphones have where 911 or rescue personnel can access only the information you have provided.)

Get in the habit of updating your medication information every two weeks or whenever you are prescribed new prescriptions or finish a round of treatment prescribed, such as penicillin or other short-term medicines.

It's crucial to keep track of all the over-the-counter supplements you're taking or have been prescribed as these may adversely affect your prescribed medicines. This is true of all prescriptions, including those prescribed by other physicians. Thus, if you are under more than one physician's care, ensure everyone is aware of the medication regime you're on.

Keep in mind that some medications may not work well with others and some supplements may have an unwanted or adverse reaction when taken during radiation or chemotherapy and may interfere with the up-take efficiency of the medicines prescribed; this includes vitamins and skin lotions. Thus, discuss this possibility with your doctors.

Your diet and eating patterns will become an essential component of your recovery and something to discuss with your physician. We'll address this in more detail in the chapter on **Creative Nutrition**.

Whenever possible, try eating more fruits and vegetables as getting nutrients and vitamins straight from the source is the best option. I recommend juicing as an alternative to soft drinks and energy drinks which are full of sugar and feed your cancer.

Your physician will typically conduct a blood test to check your B12, vitamin D, calcium, zinc and iron levels. If you're deficient in any of these, talk to your physician about options as these four vitamins and minerals will have a major impact on your health and recovery as well as help in the prevention of fatigue, anemia and osteoporosis.

Keep track of any allergies you have or develop and ensure each physician is made aware of this as not doing so can adversely affect your health and even put it at risk. For instance, I'm allergic to all kinds of adhesives; yep even the adhesives used in Band-Aids. I'm also allergic to surgical glue which many physicians use to close wounds. Allergies, regardless of how minor their effects, should be in your medical chart and on your smart phone, along with the reactions they cause. For example: hives, seizures, dizziness, etc.

When speaking to the surgeon in charge of my upcoming thyroid surgery, he stated in his parting remarks that I shouldn't worry about a scar as he was going to use surgical glue to close the incision. I promptly reminded him of my allergy to **all** adhesives. He reviewed the chart more closely and confirmed my allergy was documented. He reconsidered his typical surgical closure for thyroid surgery and used a different surgical method to suture my incision and avoid complications to my health. Thus, never assume your physician is aware of — or remembers — your allergies to medicines or material (latex, adhesives, etc.). Always point them out! As I've stated throughout this book, you are your own best advocate.

Some insurance plans have over-the-counter medication clauses/benefits which allows you to receive a set amount monthly to use for non-covered medical prescriptions and items not covered by your plan. Medicaid has this as well. They don't tell you about this so be sure to inquire. Some plans call it something different, thus check and don't take the initial, "I've never heard of that" for an answer.

Sometimes medications and supplies are covered under **durable medical equipment** or if your physician prescribes them in their **genetic** formula. (Genetic not generic.) These include items such as gauze pads, saline solution, vitamin B12, vitamin B6, vitamin C, calcium with D and Xeroform, just to name a few.

Always question your insurance provider when you are denied a prescription. Discover what they need and what form or specific technical wording they need it in to ensure payment.

Yes, the hassle is worth it when you consider that having these items covered can save you hundreds of dollars a month. Let me give you an example. Gauze pads are $6.50 for a box of 25. You'll need to change your dressing once to twice a day. If both of your breasts are affected, that's eight gauze pads a day times 30 days. That equals 240 gauze pads a month. That equates to 10 boxes of gauze pads you must purchase a month. That's $65 a month on gauze pads alone. And you'll need them for at least two months barring any complications. You're starting to get the picture, aren't you?

Warning: never allow the pharmacy or durable medical provider to give you a bag of opened gauze pads. This is unsanitary and inappropriate. You need sterile, individually wrapped gauze pads.

Request your physician write an actual prescription for these items. If they are rejected under "medical prescription," have them sent again under durable medical equipment. Yes, that is the key phrase. Xeroform, as well as lymphedema sleeves and gloves are also classified under this provision. Incidentally, you'll need a new lymphedema sleeve every six months. And though the sleeve may be a pain-in-the-ass to put on, it helps prevent lymphedema when on your arm, not in your purse. Yes, I've seen way too many women who merely walk around with their sleeve in their purse when you can see they are suffering from this disease as well.

As for Xeroform, this is a medicated gauze pad you place over your wounds to help them heal. My dermatologist recommended it for me and within a week, I began to see major improvements in the exposed sutured areas of my breasts, as well as in healing.

As with anything concerning your medical care and treatment, contact your physician. I can only share **what worked best for me** following my surgeries and the numerous complications I've experienced as I walked down this *Cancer Tamer* path. Everyone is different. Your physician should always be your number one go-to person if you have any concerns. If he or she is not helpful or clashes with you (after all we're all human) find someone else who jives better.

Some insurance companies will assign you a nurse case manager, if you have a chronic illness such as cancer. This individual is there to help you navigate the cryptic waters of medical insurance and help you with any difficulties you are experiencing in obtaining care and prescriptions. Take advantage of this service! This person will be an invaluable asset as time progresses and can be one of your best advocates.

Use the following pages to keep track of your medication and over-the-counter vitamins or supplements (prescribed or not). Remember to update them when necessary.

Allergies: (List all allergies you have including allergies to various medicines and your reaction to them. (For example, I'm allergic to Benadryl; it gives me seizures; blueberries make my lips swell; etc.))

_____

_____

_____

_____

_____

Medication: _____

Dosage: _____

Frequency: _____

Start/End Date: _____

Reason for Meds: _____

Prescribing Doctor: _____

Discontinued: _____

Reaction to Meds: _____

Notes: _____

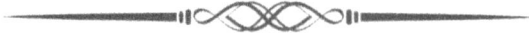

Medication: _____

Dosage: _____

Frequency: _____

Start/End Date: _____

Reason for Meds: _____

Prescribing Doctor: _____

Discontinued: _____

Reaction to Meds: _____

Notes: _____

Medication: _____

Dosage: _____

Frequency: _____

Start/End Date: _____

Reason for Meds: _____

Prescribing Doctor: _____

Discontinued: _____

Reaction to Meds: _____

Notes: _____

Medication: _____

Dosage: _____

Frequency: _____

Start/End Date: _____

Reason for Meds: _____

Prescribing Doctor: _____

Discontinued: _____

Reaction to Meds: _____

Notes: _____

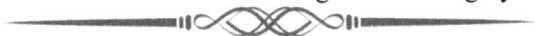
Medication: _____

Dosage: _____

Frequency: _____

Start/End Date: _____

Reason for Meds: _____

Prescribing Doctor: _____

Discontinued: _____

Reaction to Meds: _____

Notes: _____

Medication: _____

Dosage: _____

Frequency: _____

Start/End Date: _____

Reason for Meds: _____

Prescribing Doctor: _____

Discontinued: _____

Reaction to Meds: _____

Notes: _____

Medication: _____

Dosage: _____

Frequency: _____

Start/End Date: _____

Reason for Meds: _____

Prescribing Doctor: _____

Discontinued: _____

Reaction to Meds: _____

Notes: _____

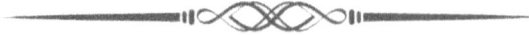

Supplements & Over-the-Counter Items:

_____

Dosage: _____

Frequency: _____

Start/End Date: _____

Reason for Meds: _____

Prescribing Doctor: _____

Discontinued: _____

Reaction to Meds: _____

Notes: _____

Supplements & Over-the-Counter Items:

_____

Dosage: _____

Frequency: _____

Start/End Date: _____

Reason for Meds: _____

Prescribing Doctor: _____

Discontinued: _____

Reaction to Meds: _____

Notes: _____

Supplements & Over-the-Counter Items:

_____

Dosage: _____

Frequency: _____

Start/End Date: _____

Reason for Meds: _____

Prescribing Doctor: _____

Discontinued: _____

Reaction to Meds: _____

Notes: _____

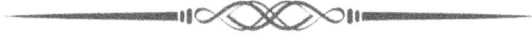

Supplements & Over-the-Counter Items:

_____

Dosage: _____

Frequency: _____

Start/End Date: _____

Reason for Meds: _____

Prescribing Doctor: _____

Discontinued: _____

Reaction to Meds: _____

Notes: _____

Supplements & Over-the-Counter Items:

_____

Dosage: _____

Frequency: _____

Start/End Date: _____

Reason for Meds: _____

Prescribing Doctor: _____

Discontinued: _____

Reaction to Meds: _____

Notes: _____

Supplements & Over-the-Counter Items:

_____

Dosage: _____

Frequency: _____

Start/End Date: _____

Reason for Meds: _____

Prescribing Doctor: _____

Discontinued: _____

Reaction to Meds: _____

Notes: _____

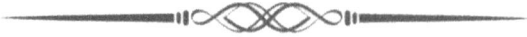

Supplements & Over-the-Counter Items:

_____

Dosage: _____

Frequency: _____

Start/End Date: _____

Reason for Meds: _____

Prescribing Doctor: _____

Discontinued: _____

Reaction to Meds: _____

Notes: _____

Supplements & Over-the-Counter Items:

_____

Dosage: _____

Frequency: _____

Start/End Date: _____

Reason for Meds: _____

Prescribing Doctor: _____

Discontinued: _____

Reaction to Meds: _____

Notes: _____

Supplements & Over-the-Counter Items:

_____

Dosage: _____

Frequency: _____

Start/End Date: _____

Reason for Meds: _____

Prescribing Doctor: _____

Discontinued: _____

Reaction to Meds: _____

Notes: _____

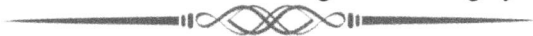

Notes:

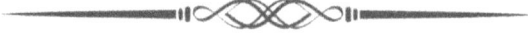

Notes:

CHAPTER 7

Cancer Tamer Posse
Organizing Your Personal Support Team

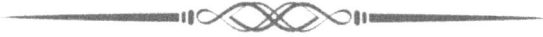

———————— ‖◦⟩⟨⟨✕⟩⟩⟨◦‖ ————————

U nlike a broken bone, getting your tonsils taken out, or passing a kidney stone, cancer does not leave you. That's not to say that it won't go into remission or be eradicated altogether. It's the aftermath of it that stays with you: the emotional turmoil, the scars, the fear of recurrence.

In the first few weeks and months after your diagnosis, you'll spend a lot of time running from one doctor's appointment to another. You'll be tested, probed and ultimately — most likely — get hit with a ray gun (radiation treatment). I call it the, "Meeting Marvin the Martian" or "Things I have in common with an alien abductee" phase of life.

And just when you think you have this insanity under control, something else crops up that throws you for a loop and leaves you wondering what happened. What to do? How to make ends meet since you've taken a lot of time off work and have more to go? If you work for yourself, you may find that you're unable to keep up with the hours you once devoted to your business to make it top notch.

On top of all that, there are the typical daily chores which still need to be performed. The house needs to be cleaned, dishes need to be washed and laundry needs to be done. Wait, did I forget those pesky things called shopping for groceries or making dinner, lunch or breakfast?

If you have kids at home or are taking care of another person (a sick or disabled child, elderly parents or a spouse) that's one more task to add to the plethora of items on your to-do list.

There's just not enough time in a day to get everything done which is true whether you're sick or not. It's a pity we don't come with clones! Personally, I'd have placed an order for two clones right up front.

So, what do you do?

Answer — you turn to family, friends, your church, your neighbors, various community resources and organizations, etc. You create your very own *Cancer Tamer Posse* to help you with it all.

In this chapter, we'll discuss how your *Cancer Tamer Posse* can help reduce your stress by performing some of those daily tasks on your list. Yes, you're still in charge; however, it's a benefit to have your *Posse* around to help pick up the slack, especially after surgery and during your recovery.

One benefit of sharing your diagnosis with family and friends is having them assist you in doing research into your condition and treatment. There's so much to learn and so many intricate facets to cancer that it can be overwhelming to try and cover it all yourself, especially when you're first diagnosed and dare I say, in terror of what will happen next.

Trust me, I've tried going it alone. I pride myself on how well I can handle anything the world can throw at me and I typically come out on top. Yet, cancer has kicked my butt a few times thus far. Having — allowing — someone in my corner is a godsend.

If you're diagnosed with more than one type of cancer at once, it becomes a nightmare to juggle it all (i.e., breast cancer, thyroid cancer, leukemia, etc.)

Let your family and friends help you in your research and recovery. Assign each individual with the task(s) you feel they are best qualified and suited for or assign them the task they may wish to take on. Even small children and teens can take a few chores off your plate. The beauty of allowing them to assist you is the sense of control they'll experience knowing they helped in some small way.

They love you; let them show it!

If you're not used to asking for help or feel vulnerable doing so, ask a family member or friend to coordinate organizing volunteers on your behalf. Explain what you need, including your preferences — it's all right to be specific in what you need done. Remember, they love and care for you and want to be of service.

Remember you can assign more than one person to each task. Or, if the person assigned can't perform the task, isn't following through as necessary or isn't the best person for the task, feel free to change things around. It's whatever you need to make life easier. Yep, I know, a million dollars would help and not having cancer would be even better, but alas, it is what it is, and you are clever enough to make it work for you. I have faith in you.

Below, I have gone into detail on a few of the more necessary tasks you will need to address during your care and recovery. I've also added additional tasks at the end of the chapter for you to consider. Feel free to add other tasks specific to your needs.

Task — Internet Research

There is a host of frightening and erroneous information out there, especially in blogs and websites which are targeting cancer patients for their products. Many use fear tactics to accomplish their sales pitch. I was lured into one of these sites shortly after my diagnosis. (A time when you're very vulnerable.)

A well-meaning friend heard of a site and recommended it without having first reviewed it himself. Though the information originally appeared very authoritative about cancer, it slowly became apparent what the ruse was. It spoke about what cancer was doing to my body and how I could overcome cancer's life-threatening effects *if only* I used their proprietary formulated supplements which cost $69.95 for a 30-day supply. The website pitch went as far as to declare that without their supplements I was looking at death in two to five years. *Bastards!*

If I could reach through my computer screen and slap them upside the head, I would have. How dare they prey on my fears like that — or anyone else's! Thus, having a friend take on the task of looking online for information is a big relief.

The American Cancer Society provides valuable information about various types of cancer and treatment options. They will send you the information via email or if, like me you prefer paper, they'll ship it to your home. You don't even have to pay postage. (Personally, I prefer paper. It's easier to access, I can take it with me to appointments, and I can scribble my notes and thoughts on the pages. It's also easier to share with others on the go.) Best of all, their trained operators are fantastic and so willing to help. They were a tremendous resource during my initial diagnosis and even after my surgery. They also will speak to family and friends who have questions. They are also a valuable resource as you enter the treatment phase of your diagnosis.

Note: There are other organizations that provide information on cancer. Find the ones that best meet your needs. Yes, you can use them all.

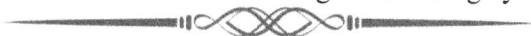

Name: _____ Number: _____
Special   Notes/Instructions:

_____

_____

_____

Name: _____ Number: _____
Special   Notes/Instructions:

_____

_____

_____

_____

Task — Handling Financial Affairs

If you don't have a spouse or partner, designate a trusted friend to maintain your finances for you while you're recuperating. For instance, have them prepare your checks for the monthly bills or contact your creditors to discuss delays in payment. I gave my creditors a heads-up on my condition which made it easier to have them refund late fees which occasionally occurred.

Your financial aid can also help pay for groceries when they're delivered or purchase them for you. You can have a separate credit card issued or purchase a pre-paid card for this purpose. You may also wish to create a power of attorney for someone to act on your behalf for a specific period of time. Once you're better and can take over the responsibility once more, you can tear up the power of attorney.

Name: _____ Number: _____
Special Notes/Instructions:

_____

_____

_____

_____

_____

Name: _____ Number: _____

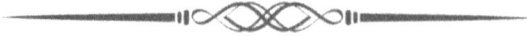

Special Notes (How would you like to help?)

_____

_____

_____

_____

Task—Dealing with the Insurance Company

Dealing with the insurance company may sometimes feel like a practice in futility. You'll soon feel like Sisyphus from Greek mythology; he's the one who must push a boulder up a hill only to have it roll over him and fall back to the bottom once more for all eternity.

It took me over seven months to obtain a customized compression sleeve to help prevent lymphedema which I eventually was diagnosed with because of the insurance company's delay.

When dealing with an insurance company, you must take yourself out of the equation and become an objective observer. Yes, at times, giving in to tears and frustration while talking to them on the phone may make them more receptive and prompt them into acting more expediently. And though it's a pain in the ass at times to deal with them, it's a necessity.

If dealing with them is not your cup of tea, you can assign your spouse, family member or friend to deal with them initially or in certain situations or hire someone (an attorney) to be your advocate. The essential point is, if you need it, you'll have to push for it — at times even fight for it. Don't despair! Each skirmish you overcome merely proves how strong you are.

Always treat yourself to something fun after you've spoken to them or accomplished your goal. Remember to write down, in your journal, the information of whom you spoke to and what is being done. If you've already spoken twice or three times to someone on the same issue, write a letter of "Protest and Concern" to the insurance coordinator. The fact that you've put your issue in writing means they have a specific timeframe — by law — to act on it — typically 15 to 30 days.

If you're merely going back and forth on the phone, as I did for my compression sleeve, everyone will repeatedly change their story to cover their ass. So, cover yours! Put it all in writing. One great thing about putting your needs and requests and issues in writing is that you don't have to constantly repeat yourself which can be extremely frustrating and insanely annoying. You can reference the letter you've written and thus get rid of the negative energy that's stressing you out. Also, having everything in writing allows you to have documentation when necessary.

As I've mentioned repeatedly, keep a notebook of all your medical and insurance transactions. Jot down every time you interact with your physicians and the various representatives of the insurance company — time, dates, phone numbers, extensions, etc. This is all crucial information.

I filled-up two composition notebooks after only nine months into this journey — my *Cancer Tamer Journey* — as I've dubbed it. I'm sure I'll have many more notebooks to fill over the years.

Let's face it, we can't remember it all; even Wonder Woman would have trouble remembering. Thus, make your life easier in every any way you can. You'll thank yourself later that you did.

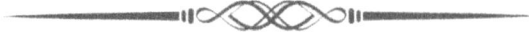

Jot down the name and number of the individual at your insurance company who is your nurse case manager, your home health aide coordinator, and their social worker so that your **Cancer Tamer Posse** member assigned to this task knows who to contact.

Nurse Case Manager: _____
Number: _____

Home Health Aide Coordinator: _____
Number: _____

Insurance Social Worker: _____
Number: _____

Name: _____ Number: _____
Special Notes/Instructions: (How would they like to help?)
_____
_____
_____
_____
_____

Name: _____ Number: _____
Special Notes/Instructions:
_____
_____
_____
_____
_____

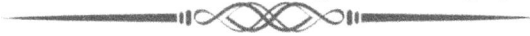

Task — Carpool

Another task which is invaluable is having a carpool. Create a list of all your family and friends who can provide you with a trip to the doctor's office when you need it — something you'll need often. You'll also need help to perform errands such as picking up medications, laundry, grocery shopping, etc.

If you have kids or teenagers at home, don't forget carpooling can also include getting them back and forth to activities or picking them up and dropping them off at school. Try to coordinate this with other parents or your children's friends in the area. This will be a major load off your shoulders.

Name: _____ Number: _____
Special Notes (How would they like to help?)

_____
_____
_____
_____
_____

Name: _____ Number: _____
Special Notes (How would they like to help?)

_____
_____
_____
_____
_____

Task — Medical Transportation

Check with your insurance company as they may provide medical transportation — most do, including Medicaid.

If you're in NYC, consider Access-A-Ride — other states may have their version of this public service as well. Access-A-Ride is an easy process to sign up for. Remind them to specify that you can bring your personal care aide (PCA) when traveling. This is essential to allow your home health aide to accompany you on appointments and on errands.

Once approved, Access-A-Ride will provide you with transportation wherever you need to go, including laundromat, grocery shopping, visiting friends, etc.

Warning: I recommend you carry a book or two with you to cope with the waiting time and delays. It's essential to carry your phone charger with you — my phone's battery always dies during every trip to the doctors. I think it's my phone's way of rebelling. You will need a working phone to coordinate pick-up with the car service while on your appointments.

On a side note, if you don't own a cell phone or can't afford one, you might qualify for the FREE cell phone provided by Medicaid. It's sometimes known as the "Obama Phone." It provides you with 250 minutes of free service and you can obtain additional minutes for a fee.

If you are a veteran, contact the VA for transportation assistance.

Another great transportation resource is the American Cancer Society through their *Road to Recovery* program. Their number is 800-227-2345. They are a phenomenal resource. Best of all, it's free!

Warning: All these programs may drive you a little crazy with their bureaucracy, their pick-up delays, and their operator complacency. I'm talking super-pissed-off crazy. However, don't let that spoil your sanity or mental health. Use them as a last resort if you don't have a car of your own or other means of transportation.

Name: _____ Number: _____
Special Notes/Instructions:

_____
_____
_____
_____
_____

Name: _____ Number: _____
Special Notes/Instructions:

_____
_____
_____
_____
_____

Task — A Shoulder to Lean On
(otherwise known as preserving your mental health)

If you find yourself depressed or overwhelmed at any time, reach out. There are organizations out there with free services. The American Cancer Society is available 24/7 at 1-800-227-2345. And the Staten Island University Hospital has a free CALM line where you can listen to a five-minute meditation recording at 1-800-226-CALM. (I'll warn you now that recording is just a little "fast" talking for my taste, but that's because if he doesn't keep talking, the system will hang up. However, it's still a great resource.)

The Department of Veterans Affairs has a 24/7 hotline 1-800-273-8255; press option 1. You don't need to be the cancer patient for these services; friends and family are welcomed as well.

As I've stated throughout this book, educate yourself and become your own best advocate. I often joke that I'm getting my life's PhD in cancer — you will as well.

Seek out organizations, community programs, family and friends that can assist you with what you need done. Sometimes, you will be surprised at where the help comes from.

On a side note, it's OK to tell friends or family members that you need a day free of cancer. They love and care for you and will repeatedly ask you about your cancer, its progress and your healthcare appointments. Sometimes, you just need to *Stop talking about it.*

Have a cancer free day, weekend or whatever time you need and enjoy. Go out to a movie, walk along the beach, listen to records — whatever you want or need. Discuss this need for "down time" with your loved ones. I'm sure you will all get a great benefit from it as you will all need a break from the stress and fears associated with your condition.

If you're married, remember to include a date night no less than once a week to enhance and maintain your intimacy. This isn't about sex. It's about solidifying the bond between you. Unfortunately, the divorce (split up) rates are high for women with breast cancer. There are many factors related to this tragedy; thus, make your relationship with your partner or love interest a priority. And remember, during date night there is no discussions about cancer. That can be done any other night.

You can also schedule a "fun night" with your children, giving them some individualized time with you, something they'll need to stay emotionally healthy.

Name: _____ Number: _____
Special Notes (How would they like to help?)

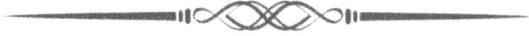
_____
_____
_____
_____
_____

Name: _____ Number: _____
Special Notes (How would they like to help?)

_____
_____
_____
_____
_____

Task — Spring Cleaning

One thing I started doing immediately after my diagnosis was a major "spring cleaning" in my home. I got rid of books, clothing, old junk that I no longer needed nor used in years and gave it away or tossed it out. It's not so much that I was being morbid and anticipating my death — though there was a little of that going on — it was more about the fact that I wanted to get my life in order and get rid of the clutter.

I got rid of everything and anything in my life that no longer fit or was taking up valuable energy. It was a form of cleansing — and it felt great!

I will admit, I'm still doing spring cleaning nine months later, getting rid of more things that don't fit the new me or my "new body" after my lumpectomy and bi-lateral breast reconstruction. Not to mention, there were some items, I didn't want my son or anyone else going through. (Insert big naughty grin here.)

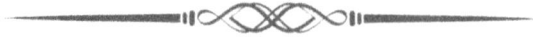

Best of all, as I went through my stuff, I not only found keepsakes I hadn't realized I had, I freed up lots of space in my closet which of course, I have since filled up with new clothing.

This "spring cleaning and cleansing" of sorts was also mentally and emotionally healthy.

Here's another incentive for "spring cleaning/cleansing": you can host a garage sale and make a few bucks. Swap things with your family and friends. This swap will come in handy as you begin to eat healthier and exercise, and the pounds fall off.

I juice and eat healthy and walk daily. This has helped me to get rid of over 49 pounds thus far. I've dropped three pant sizes, and going into a fourth (from size 18 to size 12). Instead of constantly buying new clothes, especially pants, I've been trading my larger clothes with family and friends, and it's saved me tons of money.

On a side note, you can ask your home health aide to help you with your "spring cleansing." However, she's not required to do so as that falls outside of her scope of duties. If you've got a great aide — like mine — she'll help, or you can invite friends over to help and then return the favor at their home and help them go through their closets. An added bonus when doing this is that you now get to raid their closet.

You may only be able to supervise as the work is done due to surgery constraints, medication or fatigue, but that's OK. It's a fun discovery nonetheless. You'll find yourself conducting "spring cleansing" often in the months and years ahead.

Name: _____ Number: _____
Special Notes/Instructions:

_____
_____
_____
_____
_____

Name: _____ Number: _____
Special Notes (How would they like to help?)

_____

_____

_____

_____

_____

Task — Home Health Aide

If you're like me and don't have family or friends near and don't belong to a local church or community group, discuss the need for a home health aide with your physician. I will let you know up front that your doctor's response most likely will be, "Your insurance won't pay for that."

That's not necessarily true!

Do not let them put you off. Sometimes, you or your designated advocate will need to demand and fight for services such as these. It's part of the journey.

Home health aides are typically referred to you after surgery. If you are undergoing chemotherapy prior to surgery, you can request a referral for this service.

Keep in mind, you are your own best advocate and sometimes, your only advocate.

Don't despair if you "give up" today and don't want to deal with the stupidity of things; there's always tomorrow or next week. By then, you'll have a little more energy, a little more determination and a lot more fire.

Advocating for yourself is about consistency! Don't worry if you're not "good" at it at first, trust in the fact that you'll become an expert in no time.

Never take "no" for an answer. Always check with your insurance company. Ask them specifically what's needed and then get it. You must be pro-active!

If you don't advocate for yourself (or have one of your *Cancer Tamer Posse* do it for you) you will flounder and not get all the services you need during these difficult times. I've learned this lesson the hard way. I hope that by sharing a little about my situations it helps you avoid the same pitfalls.

Doctor's offices will generally advise you that your insurance won't pay for things; however, all too often it is because they don't want to go through the aggravation of jumping through insurance hoops. Many aspects of care are in fact covered; however, you must occasionally — often — jump through a few frustrating hoops to obtain them.

For patients with Medicaid, you may find that your insurance provider will cover the expense of a home health aide so long as your primary physician or surgeon requests it and specifies your need for the same. Sometimes, your hospital's social worker can start the process for you.

The term "medical necessity" should be in their request. All your physician has to do is put in the request. The agency will send their own evaluators to assess how much time you need and if services are appropriate.

Warning: Your surgeon may state that you don't need or don't qualify for a home health aide or a medical nurse or wound specialist's assistance after surgery because you don't have surgical drains inserted.

THIS IS NOT TRUE!

Despite not having drains in your chest after surgery, you may be eligible for these services! Again, don't take "no" for an answer. You've had major surgery — yes, a lumpectomy, mastectomy, bilateral breast reconstruction are all major surgeries. You need all the help you can get!

Warning: Your doctor or his office may state a visiting nurse would submit the request for a home health aide once she has evaluated you after surgery and checked on your drains. However, if you don't have drains placed, she won't be sent which puts you in a Catch 22 (no visiting nurse, no referral).

When I called my doctor after finding myself in just this predicament, he stated I had to wait till my follow-up visit (seven days later) at which time the nurse navigator merely stated she couldn't help. Translation: she refused to help. It wasn't until two weeks after my surgery that I requested help from the hospital's social worker who completed the necessary paperwork request and got the ball rolling. Yep, I received assistance immediately after that.

If necessary, ask your primary physician when your surgeon or his office isn't helpful. It's like when you were a child — if Mom says no — ask Dad.

The key here is persistence. Though you want to *tame your cancer* and not be at war with your body, battling for your services is a skirmish you'll want to win — often!

When possible, try to arrange this evaluation before your surgery so that the visiting Nurse or nurse case manager can arrive at your home the week of or immediately after your surgery.

Having a home health aide will be a huge support, especially after surgery when you'll have difficulty with reaching, lifting, pushing, pulling and basic grooming needs. Even going to the bathroom or taking a shower will be a tremendous chore.

Warning: A little warning about home health aides. Make sure you find a good company to help you. I had to go through four agencies before we found one where the workers came on time and actually assisted me with my needs and didn't just sit on their butts or tell me they wouldn't help me do one thing or another. Ugh … very frustrating.

Instead of throwing in the towel when it gets frustrating, have your insurance company coordinator assist you in finding the right agency and the perfect aide for you.

Do not settle for half-par work. If an aide isn't working for you, or there is a personality conflict, contact the agency immediately and have the aide replaced. You don't need the stress at this point in your life, especially when you're recovering from surgery.

The hours spent with your aide are crucial to your recovery. If the agency aide cannot come during the hours you need, DO NOT compromise! Switch agencies. Otherwise, you will become frustrated and stressed, and you don't need that at this time in your life.

If the agency cannot accommodate your hours, change agencies immediately. If you agree to reduce your hours to accommodate them, you may lose your benefits altogether as the insurance company may deem you do not need them. You're the patient — they need to accommodate you — not the other way around.

Don't worry about making waves. Be honest. If the aide you received is not working out, say so. There is always another aide out there for you.

Another thing to consider when hiring an aide is their age, sex and stamina. Do you want a man or woman? Do you want young or mature? Yes, ethnicity is a factor. You don't need to feel as if you're prejudiced when asking for a certain ethnicity, sex or age — it is merely a preference and what works best for you. The aide will be in your home for several hours a day. You need someone you can get along with and feel comfortable around. You don't need further stress in your life at this time.

When interviewing my aides (yes, you can do that), I requested a mature Spanish woman who was in good shape — much like myself. Here's my reasoning: I'm in my 50s; I don't want someone young with whom I do not have anything in common. The first aide referred to me was 20 years old. She spent her time answering her Facebook and Twitter messages and expected me to feed her. She lasted two days.

As for language barriers, I didn't want someone whom I couldn't understand because it would put an additional strain on me. Though I speak English and Spanish fluently, I did receive someone who couldn't speak either, and I had to request that agency send someone else. When they stated they had no one else available, I switched agencies.

Asking that your aide is in physical shape is imperative! You want your aide to be able to perform the tasks assigned such as helping with housekeeping, preparing meals, going grocery shopping, helping you with personal care and most important, walking with you to help you get healthy after surgery.

Another aide they sent me complained of her legs hurting after just two blocks of walking with me after my surgery. She declared we couldn't walk every day — as I wanted to do to speed up my recovery — because she "just couldn't walk that much." I immediately asked for an aide who could walk without complaining as I needed to build my strength to fight off complications from my surgery and strengthen my body to overcome and prevent recurrences.

After four agencies and several comical encounters, I finally found the perfect home health aide who is mature, speaks English well and loves to walk. Plus, she's kind enough to help me go shopping for groceries as I cannot lift heavy objects such as milk cartons, nor lean over and pick things up. Yes, it's part of her duties; however, she does it with a good disposition, and that's tremendously important.

You can hire a friend or family member to act as the home health aide. They would need to go through one of the agencies and be certified to provide care; plus, they must be over 18 years of age. Having family and friends take care of you gets a little "delicate" as you may need them to perform the services and get frustrated when they don't or put you off. Yes, you can fire them; however, you still must deal with them afterward. Thus, be sure to choose wisely since you need assistance, and you don't want them sitting on their butts while you do it all yourself.

Here's another helpful tidbit — depending on the number of hours you receive, you may be entitled to receive ready-

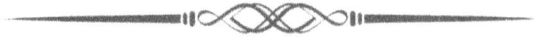

made-meals delivered to your home. Check with your insurance company and meal program organizations.

Your insurance company should assign you to a company coordinator who will follow your case and ensure you receive the benefits you need.

Yes, there's a lot to consider and try to remember as you walk this *Cancer Tamer* path. That is why I split this book on *breast cancer* into a three-part series where ***Breast Cancer: From Diagnosis to Surgery*** takes you by the hand and helps you prepare for what's ahead, what's necessary and what you may not have even considered. The second book, ***Breast Cancer: From Surgery thru Treatment,*** discusses the various aspects of care and treatment necessary and ways to stay sane while going through it all. It also will provide valuable resources you can tap into. And the final book in the series, ***Breast Cancer: Recovery & Beyond,*** will discuss how to stay focused, stay healthy and look forward to your future.

On a personal note, I'm writing these books as I am going through cancer treatment and recovery. I hope the experiences I've encountered and the tidbits I share will assist you through your own *Cancer Tamer* journey.

As ever, feel free to share your ideas and various aspects which worked well for you that we may all learn from each other. Our website is: www.CancerTamer.org and my email is info@CancerTamer.org.

Name: _____ Number: _____
Special Notes/Instructions:

_____
_____
_____
_____
_____

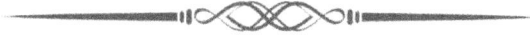
Name: _____ Number: _____
Special Notes/Instructions:

_____
_____
_____
_____
_____

Task — Daily Chores

The evil of all evils. Household chores are a bitch and seem to never get done on your best days, let alone when you're sick. Yet, daily chores must get done or chaos will soon reign and you'll find yourself standing in front of your refrigerator for long spells trying to figure out what to eat and blowing dust off your counters.

If you have kids at home, regardless of age, have them pitch in. Yes, even three- and four-year-olds can pick up their own toys. Don't feel like you must do it all. Share the responsibility; it builds character.

If you're single like me, you have no choice but to do it all yourself. However, you don't have to be the lone wolf. You can open up to family and friends, your local church, various local organizations, Veteran Affairs, etc. Let them help shoulder a little bit of the burden. It's not forever. It's just for a little while. You might find you like having others in your life and discover amazing opportunities for growth.

Contact your insurance company and discuss the situation and obtain assistance. You may need to fight for it! That's okay, just remember, you are your own best advocate. Never give up! Stand up for yourself as you would a treasured friend and demand the services you need, if it comes to that. Yes, it can be daunting, and you may feel like a broken record having to repeat yourself; yet, it's well worth the effort — you're worth the effort.

Make a list of the necessary daily chores such as cleaning the bathrooms, cooking meals, making lunches and preparing healthy snacks. For snacks, I always make a large bowl of nuts and dried fruits, mix them together, then divide them into half cup servings in plastic baggies and put them on top of my *Life Station*. I carry these snacks everywhere. They're a great energy boost, help to curb my hunger, and they're readily available. (My *Life Station* is the specially designated area in my kitchen where I keep all the healthy food and my juicer.)

Don't forget to add dusting, watering the plants and even mail duty. You can assign a friend or your spouse to go through the weekly mail for you and put aside anything you need to address immediately. The bills can be pushed to the side to address monthly; they don't have to be addressed daily. Remember, the less stress you have and the more tranquility you can generate, the better.

Below, I've added a few tasks to remind you of the typical daily chores we all need to get done. Add your own personal tasks and activities as well in the spaces provided. Feel free to attach a loose-leaf sheet or some sticky notes to this book, if necessary. There's also space for names and numbers, and your personal notes in the following pages. Remember, though you may know everyone's number by heart or have them on your smart phone, manually print their contact information here as well to allow others assisting you to access the information. Plus, you never know when your smartphone will go on the fritz.

Tasks and Activities:

- Meals
- Laundry
- Kid's activities
- Dropping off/picking up kids
- Gym (to stay healthy)

- Visits to parents or friends
- Visits to doctors' appointments
- Cleaning house
- Work duties (employer/co-workers can handle)
- Work duties (self-employed)
- Pick up medication at pharmacy
- Walking
- Fun-time out (no cancer talk)
- Helping with wound care
- _____
- _____
- _____
- _____
- _____
- _____
- _____
- _____

Name: _____ Number: _____
Special Notes/Instructions:
_____
_____
_____
_____

Name: _____ Number: _____
Special Notes/Instructions:
_____
_____
_____
_____

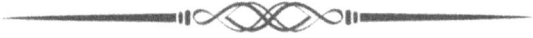
Name: _____ Number: _____
Special Notes (How would you like to help?)
_____
_____
_____
_____

Name: _____ Number: _____
Special Notes (How would you like to help?)
_____
_____
_____
_____

Name: _____ Number: _____
Special Notes (How would you like to help?)
_____
_____
_____
_____

Name: _____ Number: _____
Special Notes (How would you like to help?)
_____
_____
_____
_____

As you are discovering, there are a plethora of tasks to consider when creating your *Cancer Tamer Posse*. Once you decide which family members and friends you'd like to share your diagnosis with, discuss with them how they can best assist you in the coming weeks and months ahead.

Though you may pride yourself on your "excellent memory" and ability to care for yourself and others, cancer has a way of making your mind go blank, knocking you on your ass and backing up to roll over you once more. Having this information written down allows others to know who to call on your behalf and allows them to get the job done.

Set aside your pride, if necessary. Now is not the time to prove how strong you are — you prove that just by existing. Now is the time to allow family and friends to help and give them a sense of control; something you know is a rare commodity with this disease.

If old feelings of hurt and pain crop up, allow yourself and "them" to let those go and start anew. Letting go doesn't mean you've forgotten or forgive; it just allows you not to stay stuck.

Take a moment to divide the work up and assign your *Cancer Tamer Posse* their tasks. Be realistic when assigning tasks. Keep in mind who would be best suited for each task, has the skills and desires to perform them. Don't forget to consider time constraints. The last thing you want is to get frustrated because someone couldn't meet their assigned tasks and you were depending on them.

Be realistic!

Feel free to assign two individuals to the same task and allow them to take turns to minimize the impact on them. (Let them figure it out.)

Never forget the one simple truth so many women overlook when going through the insanity of breast cancer — **you are a smart, resourceful, vibrant spirit and you've been advocating for yourself since you were born,** from crying to be held, having your diapers changed, and getting fed, to telling someone they were being rude and inappropriate. Dealing with doctors, insurance companies and others during this time is no different. Yes, it can be challenging and seem futile at times, however, you'll have so many stories to tell about your experiences that you'll be able to write a book or star in your own comedy show.

Remember, breast cancer is merely one more bump in the road of life. How you maneuver through it is ultimately your choice.

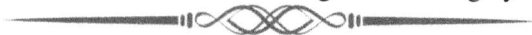

Notes:

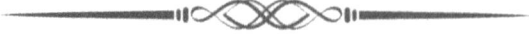

Notes:

CHAPTER 8

Creative Nutrition

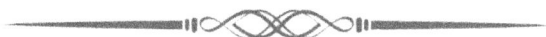

———— ||∽⟨✕⟩∾|| ————

N
o one likes to talk about dieting, so I won't mention that awful word either. Nor am I going to spout requirements on portion sizes, or worse yet, calorie counting. What I will discuss with you is nutrition or rather *Creative Nutrition* as I like to call it.

I recall the comical horror of the first time I went to see a nutritionist after I was diagnosed with breast cancer. She sat across from me digging through her desk and literally threw rubber food items at me. They were "portion size appropriate" too.

She discussed the caloric intake I was "allowed" to consume daily as well as my liquid intake — eight glasses of water — we all know that one. And yep, several more minutes of more plastic food — in combinations this time — thrown my way to ensure I had fully absorbed the correct portion sizes.

I felt like I was being assessed for gastric bypass surgery instead of being helped to identify foods which could help me eat healthier and overcome my cancer challenges, or help me detox after the radiation and chemotherapy treatments that were on the menu for the months following my surgery.

Not once did the nutritionist discuss the actual nutritional value of the foods on the list she provided nor which fruits or vegetables I should eat or stay away from. Like staying away or limiting my carrot and banana intake because of their high sugar content. Sugar — carrots? Who knew! Or that juicing is great but smoothies with lots of fruit can mean you're ingesting too much sugar which feeds your cancer. Or that not getting enough fiber can lead to diverticulitis in your colon. (Diverticulitis occurs when you get "folds" in your colon, and food, especially seeds, can be trapped in those folds and develop into health issues.)

I cringe and run in the opposite direction when someone starts talking to me about ounces or measuring cup. For me, I believe the golden rule is — or should be — eat whatever you want, just be sure it's healthy!

As for portion sizes, you know when you're over indulging. If you do so today, be good tomorrow and the rest of the week. **It's not about will power, it's about choice.** Choosing a better, healthier life for yourself every time.

Eat as many fruits and vegetables as you desire, though consider using a one to three ratio in your smoothies — one fruit with every three vegetables.

If you can buy everything organic, fabulous. If not, do what you can and stock up slowly. Throw in some protein: meats, nuts, and pumpkin or flax seeds, and you're well on your way to creating a new revolution of healthy nutrition for yourself.

Explore cookbooks and tweak the recipes to your tastes and needs. Here are a few examples: use wild rice instead of white, use raw brown sugar instead of processed white sugar. Here's a trick I use. When the recipe calls for sugar, I use half what's required. Sometimes I'll substitute honey for a more organic slant and then use only one-third of what's required in sugar. Best of all, your substitution is a healthier choice and tastes just as great.

Personally, I don't care for clover honey, but sunflower or orange blossom is delicious. Though I've discovered that when making cakes and breads, substituting honey for sugar will make it seem a little mushy, like pudding and not as "grainy." It'll still taste just as delicious, if not more so.

Hey, I'm no chef. I merely love to experiment when making my meals. *Creative Nutrition* is a blast. You'll be surprised at the delicious and healthy meals you'll soon have on your table.

In my quest to eat better, my company — the Cancer Tamer Foundation — joined forces with **Thrive Market Online** to help bring more nutritious whole foods to your table. Sign up for their program through our website. They have free memberships for low income families and veterans. They are the "Costco" of whole foods. Best of all, for every membership they receive which is made through our website link, the Cancer Tamer Foundation receives 40 percent of the membership cost which goes toward funding our FREE workshops. Review our website for further information at www.cancertamer.org/sponsors/thrive-online.

Yes, you should forego beverages such as soda, energy drinks, beer and alcohol due to their caffeine and sugar properties, not to mention all their other unhealthy ingredients. (You already know this.) On those rare occasions when you really need to let loose and get drunk, it's OK to fall off — or better yet, choose to jump off — the healthy cancer wagon. Making it a choice — **your choice** — means you take responsibility for eating and/or drinking poorly and understand that doing so may have consequences other than a simple hangover. But that's okay, we all need to do that every now and then. If you find yourself doing it often, talk to a friend or your hospital's social worker.

Don't allow yourself to get roped into the calorie counting, measuring cup craze when you see a nutritionist. You're a cancer patient. You are NOT there to lose weight!

You're there to discover how to eat healthy. The pounds will fall off as you implement healthier eating and exercise habits.

You don't have to become a crazy health freak. You do, however, need to become conscientious of what you put into your body.

I won't lie to you, it is hard — sometimes excruciatingly so — to choose healthy foods over all those gorgeous delicious looking junk foods we've grown accustomed to eating for decades. Not to mention, how much quicker and easier it is to simply hit the drive-thru at the local fast food joint or pick up a phone and dial for delivery.

You'll have to decide for yourself what's best for you in the long run and what will help you maintain or improve your health for the years ahead. Look at it this way, is the 20 minutes you saved at the drive-thru worth your physical health or delayed recovery; or worse a recurrence of cancer or its symptoms? (Nope, not trying to scare you healthy, just being honest and realistic.)

In my quest to eat healthier, I discovered the book, *Crazy Sexy Juice* by Kris Carr. In it, Kris provides many scrumptious recipes for juicing vegetables and fruits and creating smoothies as well as using nut milks. I was amazed at how fast and easy her recipes were to make, and even more so, how delicious they tasted. I found myself becoming a *mad scientist* incorporating all the different fruits and vegetables I loved into a smoothie or a juice. Best of all, every recipe was deliciously scrumptious. I devoured them quickly.

I never realized how wonderfully delicious eating healthy could taste!

Now I juice once or twice daily. Best of all, I find I'm healthier and have more energy when I juice. Yes, I have experimented with myself to determine if juicing was really helping. After juicing daily for a month, I stopped for a week and found I didn't have as much energy and my mood wasn't as vibrant. Though my decreased joyful mood could have been attributed to circumstances and complications with my recovery, once I began juicing again, I felt much better despite the complications with my health. (Mental attitude and perception is more than 80 percent of the battle.)

If you're curious about the difference between a smoothie and juicing here it is in straightforward, no-nonsense terms: Juicing takes the juice out of the vegetables as it compresses and smashes it down. The pulp is thrown into one section and the juice (liquid) is thrown into the other. Hence, all you get is the juice. When you're doing a smoothie, you're getting all the fiber of the vegetables and fruits you've mixed together. (If you are experiencing diverticulitis in your colon — again, this is where your colon folds and traps food particles — then you want to drink at least one healthy smoothie a day which will fill you with most, if not all, of your daily fiber requirements. The juices you create yourself are better than those horrible chalky tasting fiber drinks on the market. Thus, why not take the five minutes you'll spend on creating your own juice and smoothies and eat something that you'll love and is also healthy for you. Your taste buds will enjoy it and your body will love you for it.

I often joke with friends that I'm not sure if the juices and smoothies I'm creating taste great or if it's just my brain saying, "If you don't drink this you won't get healthy and you'll die — you have cancer."

Does it really matter why I (or you) think these juices taste fabulous? The fact is you're eating healthier; getting rid of unwanted weight; and, have more stamina and feel better than you have in years.

Decide for yourself how healthy you wish to become then devote some time to your goal — your choice.

I will warn you, when you start out, picking the right fruits and vegetables, reading ingredient labels and foregoing what you are accustomed to eating will be difficult. Yet, it's a challenge you are more than capable of meeting — and excelling at.

I recall I became a little obsessed with the desire to eat healthier. (I call it my crazy cancer phase.) I bought fruits and vegetables and got upset that they spoiled before I got around to eating them. That was a lot of money tossed away — money I needed for medication and health care costs.

Now, I cut up the fruits and veggies and freeze the ones I know I won't get to immediately. Freezing them actually makes my smoothies and juices so much more delicious because the fruit is cold. No need to add ice which merely dilutes the nutrition I'm trying to ingest.

You will need to decide what you're willing to give up and what you're willing to re-invent for yourself. For instance, I love salsa but every brand on the market has tons of ingredients and artificial preservatives; some even have soy in them which aren't good choices for someone with cancer. Rather than give up my love for salsa, I decided to invent my own version — without the preservatives and artificial flavors and who knows what else. Come to find out, my salsa is much better than the ones I'd been buying for years. Now family and friends have me make some for them. Best of all, it takes less than five minutes to whip it up from scratch using fresh ingredients. I add all the ingredients I enjoy like fresh onions, peppers, tomatoes and garlic to my specific tastes. When I want to go a little Tex-Mex, I even add corn. Hey, it's *Creative Nutrition* after all. The only downside I've found is that the salsa won't last long in your fridge — maybe five to seven days. But then, there's not much that wouldn't go great with a little fresh salsa. Besides, you can always add it to your tomato sauce.

Salsa isn't the only nutritious treat I've reformulated. I've also created sunflower and coconut butter fudge; I've even made my version of peanut butter chocolate cups, only I substituted almond and sunflower butter for peanut butter to make it healthier. I also ensured the chocolate I buy doesn't contain soy. Ironically, I've never cared for chocolate; however, these little creations are scrumptious, and family and friends love them. (Yep, I'm getting them to eat healthier as well.)

I'll warn you, it's virtually impossible to find chocolate without soy. However, Nestlé® Toll House Dark Chocolate morsels have 53 percent cacao and no soy. Some of their other brands do contain soy, thus, be sure to read the labels carefully.

As you may already know, soy is an estrogen-based product, and if you have been diagnosed with estrogen positive/reactive breast cancer, soy and anything that contains soy is something you want to stay far away from.

Warning: Soy is in almost everything we eat, including many energy bars. Read the labels carefully!

I recommend you find recipes you like and make them your own. Substitute where necessary to make it a healthier meal. And most of all, be creative! I've made some weird concoctions to date like pumpkin chili and using my apple lime bits as makeshift dipping spoons for my guacamole.

Be playful.

Cooking is a fun way to express your creativity.

Whenever possible, eat more fruits and vegetables as getting nutrients and vitamins straight from the source is the best option. Consider juicing as an alternative to soft drinks and energy drinks which are full of sugar and feed the cancer.

Don't worry if a few of your nutritious creations are a little too "exuberant." That's okay. Just don't make that dish again. Try other ingredients which will make it taste better. I do that with juices all the time.

For instance, if I don't particularly like a juice I've made, I'll add in an apple which dilutes the original taste. If it tastes bland, I sprinkle in a little Himalayan sea salt to liven it up and make it a bit tangier. Or if I want a more healthy shakes, I'll add in some hemp chai seeds or peanut/almond butter for a little extra protein. Whatever I'm in the mood for.

Explore.

Experiment.

Create.

Get yourself a few cookbooks and re-tweak those recipes to make them healthier. I'm no expert at cooking nor on nutrition, thus, I'll leave that information to others to explain to you. However, I've taught myself what's healthy and what's not. It's a learning game which is always ongoing as there's so much to discover. This is one game you want to excel in!

As I've only been cooking for the past six months and before that my idea of a great meal was five minutes or less in the microwave, I'll be the first to point you in the direction of a cookbook. One cookbook I highly recommend is *Crazy Sexy Kitchen* by Kris Carr. (Yep, her again — do so love her recipes.) This book is one I'm using to plan meals from. Another book I purchased at the checkout counter was *Better Homes & Gardens Special Interest Publications 100 Best Pumpkin Recipes*. I must admit, I love love love pumpkins, and I've made over half the recipes in that book already. Yes, I have re-tweaked a few to my individual tastes and dietary needs.

I've even had my home health aide send me a few recipes she's found on the internet which have made for very interesting and creative dishes. My family and friends joke that I've turned my home into *Little House on the Prairie* as I'm now known for making my own homemade salsa, seasonings, even specialty olive oil.

When I cook, I'm taking responsibility for my health. I affirm my desire to become healthier and overcome cancer and its various complications. It's me loving myself! With every juice or smoothie I blend-up, with every meal I prepare, it's one more affirmation, one more way I show **myself** that I value my life and want to be around to live it to the fullest.

I'll admit, at first, I found cooking and juicing difficult and time consuming — especially since I'd never really put any effort into my cooking nor liked being in the house before. My son quips that I didn't cook this good for him growing up.

Cooking has quickly become a joy and one way for me to battle cancer. Now, not cooking for myself or thinking of eating out is distasteful. Over time, this may become the same for you.

If you want to obtain a nutritional evaluation, I recommend making an appointment with an integrative functional medicine practitioner or a naturopathic physician. They not only assess what you're eating, they can conduct special blood tests which evaluate the levels of specific vitamins and minerals in your bloodstream. Once the results are in, they can help you establish a nutritional plan that is perfect for your specific needs. And though the goal is not weight loss, getting to a healthy weight for your body type will help you *tame your cancer* and overcome health difficulties.

Below, I've shared a few of the recipes I've created along the way. Feel free to tweak them as you wish. I invite you to share your thoughts and your own recipes with us at www.CancerTamer.org/creative-nutrition.

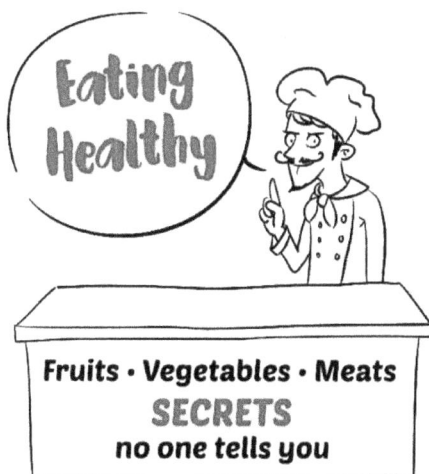

As you begin to eat healthier, keep track of your daily moods and energy level. On a scale of one to five, how much energy do you have daily? Only you can figure this out through mindful observation. Notice if your mood and energy improve as you begin eating and drinking healthier. Do you feel more rejuvenated? Do you sleep better? Do certain foods give you a better outcome or make you feel exhausted or depressed? Then plan and eat accordingly.

It's sometimes difficult to know what to eat, what amounts to consume, and whether or not those fruits and vegetables are truly healthy or merely empty calories that will exacerbate your condition.

It's even more difficult to remember which fruits and vegetables you should buy organic and which are OK to purchase "regular." There are several websites and books which provide you with a list; however, one of the best ways to remember is based on the "skin" the item has. For example, oranges have a thick skin, thus, most of the pesticides used will remain on the outer layer of the skin and are easily removed when you peel it. Thin skinned vegetables and fruits such as apples and cucumbers can hold pesticides and chemicals on their skin despite being washed. Thus, it's best to purchase the organic variety or use a peeler and take the skin off.

Below are a few recipes which have worked for me as well as information I've discovered along my Cancer Tamer journey.

Juice & Smoothie Recipes to Consider

If you're like me and love your smoothies and juices cold, consider juicing your veggies beforehand. Simply run them through your juicer, and pour the juice into an ice cube tray. Once frozen, place those ice cubes into a plastic bag and keep them in your freezer till you're ready to use them. When you're running late or low on energy, just grab a handful of fruit/veggie ice cubes and toss them into your blender. Add a cup or two of almond milk (or your nut milk of choice) and you're ready to go. This not only has you creating some wonderful veggie/fruit combinations, it keeps them from spoiling. Remember to label your baggies since some ice cubes look alike.

When creating juices, add a peeled apple if you are not thrilled with the taste. This will help neutralize the flavor and allow you to change it up a bit. Create your own combinations as you go along. The way I see it, you can't go wrong when combining the fruits and vegetables you love. Freeze any leftover juices in an ice cube tray to use in your future smoothies. You can also freeze fresh bananas to thicken your juices and ensure a cold icy drink. (Be sure to peel the banana before freezing it.)

Personally, I use a Breville Juice Fountain which is mid-range in price at about $170. I've also used a Hamilton Beach Big Mouth Pro Juicer which costs about $70. You want to spend the extra $10 to get the pitcher to catch your creations. I purchased one without the pitcher and had spilled juice everywhere.

Each juice recipe below makes approximately one serving. Double the recipe to share with family or friends or to create extra for later. Keep them in an airtight container to preserve their nutrients. Add a tablespoon of flax seeds, pumpkin seeds, or chia powder for an additional energy boost. Adding a spoonful of almond butter or sunflower butter tastes great, too, and is a great source of protein.

It typically takes approximately five to fifteen minutes to prep and make your juice. I prefer to peel my apples, cucumbers, and carrots or any fruits or vegetable with a thin skin. Core your apples and tightly pack your kale or spinach before adding it to your juicer machine. Personally, I prefer Granny Smith apples because they're a little tart; however, you can use any apples you enjoy most. The size of the fruits in these recipes should be medium or larger.

Juices

The prep time to make the juices and smoothies as well as mixing them is approximately five to seven minutes. I recommend peeling fruits and vegetables with thin skins and taking the pits out prior to using them. For aesthetics, I use wine glasses or fun designer cups and glasses since we are all visual human beings and eating and drinking something that looks good makes it that much more pleasurable. Blend all the ingredients in your juicer. Note, you'll want to wrap your kale and spinach tightly so it doesn't fly into the pulp shoot. And sprinkle the salt after juicing.

Morning Monster
2 Granny Smith apples
1 cucumber
1 navel orange
1 kiwi
1 cup of kale or spinach

Two of Six
1 navel orange
1 Granny Smith apple
2 celery stalks
2 fat cucumbers
4 carrots
1 head of lettuce
A sprinkle of Himalayan sea salt (optional)

Smoothies

When creating your smoothies, any high-powered blender will do. Don't worry about purchasing fancy smoothie makers, they're typically just as good as the blender you already have. When the recipe calls for ice cubes, this is where you use the previously juiced fruits and vegetables you froze. Keep in mind that if you're using the entire fruit in your blender, you will keep all the pulp and your smoothie will be thick.

A quick note about dairy milk versus nut milk: the reason you repeatedly hear about the need to limit or completely eliminate dairy products from your diet is because of all the antibiotics, hormones and chemicals pumped into cows. These same chemicals then toxify our bodies when we eat or drink these products. Therefore, seek out dairy products which contain no antibiotics or hormones. I'll warn you, these products can be a bit expensive. Whenever possible, swap nut milk for dairy.

One trick to making your smoothies cold without adding ice is to freeze your fruits and bananas. (Be sure to peel the banana first before freezing.) Adding a frozen banana to all the juices below will make your smoothies thicker and delicious. You can also add yogurt and protein powders for more nutrition. Feel free to substitute fruits or veggies as you wish.

China's Favorite
1 cup of almond milk (milk of your choice)
2 medium carrots
1 cup of pineapples
1 cup of strawberries
1 cup of kale or spinach
1 frozen banana

Sunrise Surprise
1 cup of cantaloupe
1 cup of carrots
1 cup strawberries
1 cup almond milk
1 tablespoon almond butter (great for added protein)
1 frozen banana

Coconut Delight
1 cup coconut water
1 cup almond milk
1 cup strawberries
2 tablespoons almond butter
1 frozen banana

Snacks to Quiet the *Craving Monster*

Who doesn't love snacking on something delicious between meals? After a long day running from one doctor's appointment to another, it's always a nice treat to make yourself a quick snack to relieve your hunger, especially if a full meal is too taxing to make at the moment.

Nuts make the perfect snack! They're full of protein and taste delicious. I purchase the big jugs of unsalted nuts at Costco every two weeks and prepare my own "trail and fruit mix" throughout the week.

I carry two bags of nuts in my purse and stash another in the messenger bag I always carry. Plus, I leave another in my car. You never know when you'll be hungry. These nut mix baggies are perfect for holding the *craving monster* at bay. Not to mention, they add the necessary protein needed to help you heal after surgery.

As a cancer patient, you will need to find healthy sources of protein to support your healing, especially after surgery. I was told I needed to eat sixty grams of protein a day to help me heal from my bilateral reconstruction and lumpectomy surgery — that's a lot of protein. I don't always accomplish that — and I'm not a boxer or bodybuilder so eating raw egg whites isn't on my menu; however, I do what I can. Your nutritional needs will vary, therefore, consult a nutritionist or an integrative functional medicine specialist for your dietary needs before surgery, as well as after.

Beware of any dried fruits that indicate "natural flavors" or have preservatives. Your best bet is to make your own dried fruits in a dehydrator or purchase them from a whole foods store. You don't need added toxins in your body.

Below are a couple of great recipes which take approximately five to 15 minutes to prepare, and you can eat anytime day or night. Best of all, you can prep them the day before or take them with you to your appointments and snack on them throughout the day.

Nut Mix

Though purchasing a ready-made trail mix is easier, I prefer to make my own mixes. This allows me to control the amount of dried fruits I add as well as the types of nuts used. Best of all, there is no soy, artificial favors, nor preservatives in the dried fruits which go into my mix. (Yes, some nut mixes do contain soy. If you're cancer is estrogen positive, you want to avoid soy in all your foods.)

Below is the recipe for my favorite nut mix. Feel free to add your own fruits and nuts to the mix in the quantities you desire. Toss the ingredients into a large bowl, mix well, then ladle half a cup of the nut mix into a plastic baggie. This recipe will make enough for approximately seven baggies.

Prep time: approximately five minutes

2 cups of nuts
1 cup pistachios
1 cup sunflower seeds
1 cup pumpkin seeds
1 cup dried cranberries
1 cup raisins (golden or black/or a mixture of each)
1 cup dried papaya (cut into small cubes)

Feel free to add shredded coconut or sesame sticks as well as hot spicy peanuts or wasabi peas. This is your nut mix, make it what you desire.

Because your nut mix has no preservatives, it will not keep as long as store bought bags. Not to worry, you'll devour it in no time. I make six to seven half cup baggies at a time and toss them into my handbag. They're a great source of protein which helps in your recovery. They're also a fabulous resource to kill those mid-day munchie cravings without adding unwanted sugar which feeds the cancer.

Guacamole

Avocados are a great healthy source of fat. Yes, you need fat in your diet. Avocados help you maintain lubrication in your vaginal area to avoid discomfort during sex or those pesky pelvic examines. Plus, they are a great source of "trans-fats," so eat up.

Below is a quick recipe for the best guacamole you've ever tasted. The trick to making the best guacamole is to purchase an avocado that's just a little soft when squeezing. I like the small ones which are sweeter and have more flavor. They skin is typically dark green or blackish in color. If they're hard, you can leave them out on the counter for two to three days until they ripen. If they're soft and you don't plan to eat them right away, stick them in the fridge for up to two days. Longer than that and they'll start going bad inside. If the avocados are too soft or squishy, they are too ripe and you'll want to avoid those. Also, if the inside is light yellow and hard, it's not ready. If the opposite is true or the inside is brown or gray, the avocado is no good.

Prep time: approximately 10 minutes.

Begin by peeling the avocado and removing the outer skin and pit. Cut the following ingredients into small, diced pieces and add to your avocado.

½ tablespoon minced garlic
¼ cup diced onions
¼ cup diced peppers (get colorful—yellow, red, orange)
6-8 sweet cherry tomatoes, diced (any tomato is fine)

Squeeze in half a lime. The lime juice will help make the avocado softer to mash. Add salt and pepper to taste. Once all the ingredients are added to the bowl, mash them up and mix well.

Use as much or as little as you wish of any ingredient. I always change a recipe to my personal tastes and you should too. If you like your guacamole a little chunkier, add a little more peppers, tomatoes or onions. I typically put about one-quarter cup (handful) of each. Keep in mind you want your guacamole a little chunky, you don't want to overwhelm it. If it seems the onions, peppers and tomatoes have taken over, add another avocado to the mix. You just can't go wrong with this recipe.

As for what to use to scoop up that delicious guacamole you just made, I found organic veggie or corn chips are great. (Take care with products like corn, carrots or starches as these foods turn into sugar, and cancer thrives on sugar. Thus, limit these items in your diet.)

Recently, I discovered that apple lime slices (recipe below) are a scrumptious and nutritious means to eat guacamole. I use Granny Smith apples. It's not merely delicious, it's filling as well. Best of all, you can spread guacamole on any dish to enhance it such as hamburgers and meatloaf. Yum heaven!

Apple Lime Slices

I discovered this recipe by accident when I was looking for a way to keep the apple slices from browning once I cut them up and put them in the fridge. Lime works best as lemon will make the apple taste funny, and you may not like it at all. Of course, lime and lemon are a personal taste preference.

This recipe is delicious; best of all, it's great for your heart as apples help with circulation and have been linked to helping prevent cancer.

I prefer to use Granny Smith apples as they're not too sweet, and the lime brings out their tarty goodness. Add a little Himalayan sea salt to give it a tangy flavor.

I've become very health conscious since my diagnosis so I peel my apples after I wash them with water to minimize any pesticide residue. Peeling them also allows the apple to better absorb the lime juice.

Once peeled, core your apple (take out the center with the pits/seeds). Slice the apple into bite-sized pieces or long slices. Place in a bowl and squeeze in half a lime. Sprinkle sea salt to taste and enjoy. Prep time is approximately five minutes

A Full Meal

I don't know about you but I love love love me some pumpkin pie! That delicious aroma when it's cooking, especially if you add cinnamon to it. I even enjoy watching it bubble up in the pot. Not only is pumpkin good for you with over 197 percent RDA of vitamin A and 394 mg of potassium in every cup, it tastes so damn scrumptious. Plus, it's only 30 calories per cup serving. As pumpkin is not a starch, you don't have to worry too much about the sugar content though there are 3.2 grams of sugar in each cup (according to internet statistics).

Pumpkin is part of the squash family so you can always swap winter squash, butternut squash or other types of squash if necessary. And, of course, winter squash and small pumpkins have their own healthy flavors.

Below are three of my favorite recipes. I'm no world chef. I basically toss things together that I love and make a meal out of it. As ever, feel free to alter the recipes to your individual tastes and needs.

Pumpkin & Italian Spinach Sausage

Prep time: approximately 10 minutes
Cooking time: approximately 20 minutes
Makes 3-4 servings

2 tablespoons olive oil
2 small scallop onions diced
2 small red and orange peppers diced
1 package of Italian sweet sausage with spinach
(6 sausage links sliced into round ¼ inch pieces)
2 cups pumpkin pieces, sliced in bit size chucks (you can use butternut squash — or sweet pumpkins or acorn squash — any variety of pumpkin)
1-1½ tablespoon seasoning, (mixture of: salt, pepper, rosemary, oregano, dill, basil, crushed red peppers)
1 cup pumpkin juice (if you don't have this, use vegetable stock)
2 cups each zucchini and butternut squash noodles (if only one is available, use butternut squash)

In pan, start by sautéing the first three ingredients until onions are translucent. Add in the 2 cups of pumpkin pieces, 1 tablespoon seasoning and the ½ cup of pumpkin juice. Cover and sauté for 10 minutes until pumpkin pieces are tender, and you can stick a fork in easily. Do not allow them to become too tender since you have more time for them to continue cooking.

Add in the Italian sausages and cook another 5 to10 minutes until sausages done. Add more pumpkin juice if necessary. You want a little sauce in the pan.

In a separate pan, toss in the 2 cups of zucchini and butternut squash and the remaining pumpkin juice and warm the noodles. You don't want them too mushy. Place the noodles on the plate and spoon the sausage and pumpkin bits over the noodles. This ranks a top score of five out of five on my Yummy scale.

Pumpkin Chili

Prep time: approximately 15 minutes
Cooking time approximately 25-30 minutes
Makes 4-6 servings

2 tablespoons olive oil
3 cloves garlic
½ cup mix of onions and peppers (red, yellow & orange)

In an 8-quart pot, sauté the first three ingredients above until the onions are translucent (light and a little soft). Mix and stir them frequently to keep from sticking.

Add the following ingredients:
1 tablespoon sea salt
1 tablespoon black pepper
½ tablespoon oregano
1 12-ounce can tomato sauce
1 12-ounce can chopped tomatoes
(In lieu of canned tomatoes, add 3 to 4 cups fresh cherry or grape tomatoes, as they're sweeter. Cut these tomatoes into fourths. You can use any other fresh tomatoes you like.)

3 large potatoes cut into bite size chucks
2 cups pumpkin

(About 20 pieces. Cut into 2-inch squares. They will shrink as they're cooked.)

Cook for approximately 20 minutes on low and check often. Once you can stick a fork easily into the potatoes and pumpkin, the chili is ready to eat. Feel free to add additional seasoning to your desired taste. Make this recipe you own.

Adding meat:
I'm a happy carnivore thus I need meat in my chili and love love eating steak and other meats. I do try to purchase them with as little or no hormones or free range as possible. Yes, this is a bit more expensive, but I'm worth it — and so are you.

In a separate pan, brown one pound of ground beef and season to taste. Cook thoroughly. Drain the excess oil and fat and then add the ground beef to the chili. In lieu of ground beef use chicken or ground turkey.

When browning your meat, pour 2 spoons of oil and a handful of onions and red and orange peppers in your skillet. Add a tablespoon of chopped garlic. Sauté ingredients, mixing often until the onions turn translucent. Add your favorite seasoning and allow meat to cook. I like to pour in ¼ cup of vegetable broth to help the meat cook without burning.

Seasoning: mix together 1 tablespoon of each of the following: oregano, black pepper, and Himalayan sea salt; ½ tablespoon of rosemary and onion powder; plus, a shake or two of red peppers — 3 shakes if you enjoy a kick to your meat.

Be careful not to cook the chili too long or the potatoes and pumpkin will dissolve into the chili and thicken it. That's okay, too; if it happens, you'll still enjoy the flavor.

Top with sour cream and cheddar cheese (optional). Use multi-grain crackers or corn chips to scoop it up and enjoy.

Stir Fry

I do so enjoy stir fry. It's a quick and easy nutritious dish which leads to amazing combinations of ingredients you can toss together to make a delicious meal.

As I previously mentioned, *Creative Nutrition* is all about bringing together the ingredients you enjoy most and creating a fun, tasty meal. As a cancer patient, it behooves you to discover how to eat healthier and create meals which will keep you motivated as well as promote healing.

Prep time: approximately 10 minutes
Cooking time: approximately 20 minutes

For this stir fry version, we'll add the following ingredients. As always, feel free to add or substitute any ingredients you wish. Of course, if you're a vegetarian, feel free to add other sources of protein such as beans and nuts in lieu of meat.

1 pound of beef or chicken
1 cup pumpkin pieces
1 cup Brussels sprouts (sliced or quartered)
2 cups butter squash noodles
¼ cup Granny Smith apple cut into small pieces to give the dish a little sweetness.

To start, add 2 tablespoons of olive oil to a skillet with a handful of onions and green and red peppers (¼cup of each). You can add banana (yellow) or orange peppers which are sweeter flavored. It's fun to have a colorful meal. Once the onions are translucent, add the meat.

Add your seasoning to the meat and allow it to cook for about 5 minutes before adding ½ cup of pumpkin and a ¼ cup of Granny Smith apples (optional). A half cup of Brussels sprouts sliced or quartered will add Vitamin C, potassium and iron to your meal.

If you're not using meat, consider adding half a can each of kidney and garbanzo beans for the necessary protein. Stir in ¼ cup of vegetable broth and mix ingredients. Cover for another 10 to 15 minutes, stirring occasionally. Once the meat is cooked, add 2 cups of butternut squash noodles and let steam for another 5 minutes. Mix all ingredients together and serve.

Dessert

No meal would be complete without a delicious dessert. Just because we have cancer doesn't mean we can't indulge our sweet tooth. Below is a delightful dessert of both fruits and chocolate. As I previously mentioned, the Apple Lime Slices are fantastic and very filling. They are not only great as a snack but also as a dessert. If you have the energy to create a dessert which takes a bit more time, try my version of the "peanut butter cup."

Keep in mind if you were diagnosed with estrogen positive breast cancer you will want to ensure the chocolate chips you use do not contain soy. Nestlé® Toll House Dark Chocolate morsels have 53 percent cacao and no soy. I'm sure there are other chocolate brands on the market which do not contain soy as well.

Sunflower/Almond Butter Chocolate Cups

I'll be the first to admit that I don't really care for chocolate. This may be because I'm allergic to soy and most chocolates are full of soy. However, this recipe is so deliciously decadent (and has no soy), you'll find yourself making it often.

Prep time: approximately 20 minutes

Cooking time: approximately 20 minutes
You'll need the following ingredients to make the sunflower and almond butter filling:

1 cup sunflower butter
1 cup almond butter
¼ cup honey
1 tablespoon coconut oil
1 teaspoon vanilla
½ teaspoon sea salt

Mix the ingredients well and place in the fridge while you prepare the chocolate.

Prepare a mini-muffin tray that holds 24 paper cups. Once done set aside.

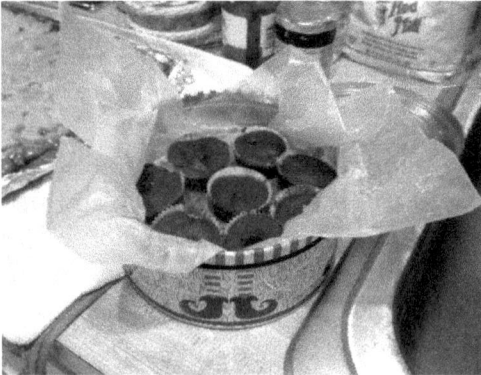

Use a double boiler to melt the chocolate. If you don't have a double boiler, use one small sauce pan to boil the water and one pan or non-plastic mixing bowl that can comfortably sit over the bowling water where you'll begin melting the chocolate, at a quarter bag at a time.

Once the chocolate is melted, pour at least ½ to 1 teaspoon into the mini-muffin cups. Use a toothpick to ensure the chocolate coats the bottom of the muffin cups. You don't want to fill the entire muffin cup with chocolate. You merely want to coat the bottom.

Once you've filled the muffin cups with the first layer of chocolate, drop 1 teaspoon of the sunflower/almond coconut mixture into the muffin cup. Use the toothpick to settle the sunflower mixture into the cup, then pour another teaspoon of chocolate over the top. Once again, you can swirl the chocolate with the toothpick.

Place the mini-muffin tray in the refrigerator for 1 hour to allow sunflower/almond chocolate cups to set. Once done, I keep mine in a tin can in the fridge. You'll want to use one or two paper cups as they can get a bit oily underneath.

They will last 1 to 2 weeks in the refrigerator.

Sesame & Sunflower Nut Bar

Just because you've been diagnosed with cancer doesn't mean you can never eat sugar or sweet snacks again, though, you do want to restrict their intake. Here's a quick recipe that's delicious and healthy with just a touch of sugar and honey. You can add various nuts to the mix to suit your tastes. Also, I found that if you toast your nuts beforehand, it'll taste better than not toasting them at all. Yes, toasting does add about 5 extra minutes to your preparation, but taste this delicious cannot be rushed. (To toast your nuts, place them in a skillet, turn the heat to medium, and stir. Do not add oil or butter. There's no need. As the nuts cook, their natural oils will release. When you hear them start to pop and the nuts begin to brown, remove them from the stove and set aside.)

You will need the following items for this recipe: wax paper, non-stick spray (optional), rolling pin, skillet and butter knife.

Prep time: approximately 10 minutes
Cooking time: approximately 20 minutes

Prepare two sheets of wax paper approximately 1 foot long. Spray with non-stick spray (non-soy) and place to the side. You don't need the non-stick spray once you get the hang of making this treat. Just be sure to lift up the wax paper slowly as it sometimes tend to stick to the mixture.

Mix together the following ingredients:
1 ½ cup sesame seeds
1 cup sunflower seeds
½cup pumpkin seeds
½ cup sliced almonds
1 cup oats (optional/see notes)

In a small pan or metal cooking bowl, bring the sugar and honey to a boil.
3 tablespoons of honey
3 tablespoons of raw brown sugar

You want the sugar and honey to melt and bubble. Once bubbling, pour the mixture over the toasted seeds. Mix thoroughly until all the seeds are saturated with sugar/honey mix. You'll want to mix quickly as the mixture will start to stick to your bowl.

Once completely mixed, pour seed mixture onto the first sheet of wax paper then place the second piece of wax paper over the top. Use the rolling pin to flatten the mixture until it is a½-inch high.

Once flattened, press the edges of the mixture in to form a square.

Let cool for five minutes then cut with knife or pizza cutter into 2-by-2- inch square bars before mixture cools completely and begins to harden. (Run the knife or pizza cutter down the mixture from left to right, then up and down to form the squares.)

Let cool for approximately five more minutes then pull off wax paper and enjoy. To harden the bars, place them on a cookie sheet and refrigerate for ½ hour. Once done, peel from wax paper and place into plastic baggies or put into decorative tin cans. Keep refrigerated. They can last in your frig for approximately 2 weeks. Take them with you for a daily pick-me-up. When not refrigerated they will get soft. That's OK, they're delicious either way.

Make It Even Healthier

Turn this recipe into an energy bar by adding a handful each of goji berries, dried cranberries, even raisins. No need to increase the honey/sugar mixture.

Experiment with the recipe and make it your own. You can't go wrong. These little energy bars are addictive. You'll find yourself making this recipe often. Don't be surprised if your kids and friends love it, too.

As you can see, cooking healthy can be fun and doesn't require much time — at least no more time than your average meal. Do a little research on the internet for recipes on the foods you enjoy most. Create your own recipes mixing together the fruits and vegetables you love. Substitute honey for sugar or reduce the sugar required in your recipes by half. I've discovered that cutting back on the sugar doesn't affect the recipe and allows me to enjoy the meal more.

Allow yourself to be creative with your nutrition.

Experiment.

Be playful.

If it's not quite what you wanted, that's okay, you'll do better on your next try as you continue to experiment and

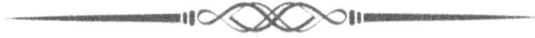

create meals for yourself. Use the space below to jot down a few of your treasured favorites.

Jot down your own *Creative Nutrition* recipes below.

CHAPTER 9

Questions to Ask Your Doctors
BEFORE Surgery

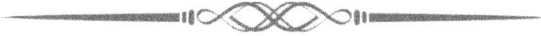

O ne of the most important things to keep in mind when you're diagnosed with cancer is that you have a right to ask questions!

You also have a responsibility to take part in your treatment options and advocate for yourself.

It's perfectly understandable and acceptable to be terrified of what will happen next and to question your own mortality; however, do not allow that fear to stop you from caring for yourself and your present and future health.

You don't have to be a doctor nor hold a PhD in cancer to ask questions; you merely need to ask them. If you're like me, you'll go out and conduct your own research on your cancer diagnosis and become familiar with its nuances. Yes, this can be a bit mind boggling and exhausting — even scary; yet what's the alternative? Do you want to be uninformed and feel powerless and helpless as strangers and well-meaning loved ones make the decisions for you? Is that really how you want to live your life?

Asking questions will provide you with a sense of control and alleviate some of the fear. Just because you don't understand the intricacies of medicine and oncology, doesn't mean you can't make informed decisions. You can! Arm yourself with knowledge and take back the power and inner strength you feel you've lost when you heard the doctor say, "You have cancer."

A great resource for questions to ask is the American Cancer Society. In their pamphlets on breast cancer, there is a whole host of questions to ask which you can use as a springboard to help you ask more of your own.

Below are a few questions I asked when I was first diagnosed with breast cancer. I expanded these questions when less than a year after my breast cancer diagnosis, I was diagnosed with thyroid cancer. Use them as a guideline to help you start a dialogue with your medical personnel, including your breast surgeon, plastic surgeon, nurse navigator and others. Add your own questions to the mix in the pages provided and jot down their answers.

I always recorded my sessions with the doctors — especially when asking questions — so that I could remember what they said. I typically played the recording back the days and weeks after so I could help alleviate my fears with their answers.

At times, my questions prompted more discussions. I was pleased that most of my physicians and the nurse navigator were willing to answer the plethora of questions I posed and help put my fears to rest. When a physician refused to do so, I'd find a new one.

Remember, you are entitled to a second — even a third — opinion. This is true of your breast surgeon and plastic surgeon; who are not always the same person. Don't feel like you must settle for the first opinion, especially if you don't agree with the treatment options provided.

The questions below are from my own personal experience and are not meant as medical advice. They are provided to give you a starting point of what to ask and as thoughts and concerns you should be aware of. As you and your loved ones conduct your own research, feel free to add your questions to the list.

The questions below are not in any specific order. Feel free to substitute breast cancer questions for questions concerning other parts of your body such as ovarian and thyroid cancer — or prostate cancer, if you're a man. Use the questions as a guide and add them to the ones you already have.

- What type of breast cancer do I have? (Estrogen/progesterone/HER 2 Neu. This is determined during the biopsy.)

- Am I positive for the BRCA1 or BRCA2 gene? Are there any other genes which would make me susceptible to breast or other cancers? (This is determined by genetic testing. Before you consider a mastectomy or ovary removal, you should have this evaluation conducted. It's simple, merely a blood test and mouth swab. They will also obtain a family history of breast cancer and other types of cancers which may run in your family.

  It's imperative to remember that if your tests are positive for the BRCA1 or BRCA2 gene, **this does not mean you will eventually have breast cancer,** if you don't have it already. It simply means, you are more susceptible to it and need to watch your nutrition, exercise, and maintain good health.)

- Can you conduct a genetic test to determine if radical surgery or medical treatment is necessary? (i.e., mastectomy and ovarian removal and/or hysterectomy)

- Is the cancer contained in the ducts or has it spread out into surrounding tissue?

- How large is my tumor? Is it growing? (You can discover the size of your tumor from the preliminary examinations — sonogram, MRI, etc.)

- What stage of cancer do I have? (Typically, you won't be "staged" until after the tumor is removed. However, you can have a preliminary stage based on the size of your tumor and its severity.)

- If I choose a dual mastectomy and ovary removal as opposed to the less invasive lumpectomy with/out reconstruction, will doing so be better for my health?

- Can I speak with a plastic surgeon about options? (mastectomy, lumpectomy, reconstruction, etc.)

- Will the breast surgeon/plastic surgeon be able to save my nipple(s) during surgery?

- Will an Oncotype DX Test be performed? If not, why not? (Note: sometimes Stage I breast cancer is not tested. However, you should request this test as it will help determine your score on the cancer scale and whether adjuvant chemotherapy — drug therapy/medication — will be beneficial for you; and if so, to what degree.)

Sometimes adjuvant therapy (aromatase inhibitors and tamoxifen) can cause more damage to your body and your quality of life than the cancer did. Therefore, you will want to assess the risk factors and determine if the risks are worth it.

- Is there time to wait to conduct surgery to allow me to fully weigh all the options and obtain other opinions or must surgery be performed immediately? If surgery is needed immediately, explain why?

- Can the breast surgeon and plastic surgeon recommend other surgeons for a second/third opinion? (Do not use physicians in the same practice for a second opinion — you want to obtain an unbiased one.)

- Once surgery is conducted, who will I be able to see for a second opinion on my treatment regime and care, if I am not satisfied with the course of treatment being taken?

  (NOTE: This question is essential as other surgeons will refuse to see you — even for a consultation — once surgery has been performed. The reality is, no one wants to step in someone else's crap. Thus, be sure the breast surgeon and plastic surgeon have a colleague you can see if necessary.)

- If the breast cancer is hormone receptor estrogen or progesterone positive, should adjuvant therapy start before or after surgery?

- Is chemotherapy or radiation necessary prior to surgery to reduce the size of my tumor? What benefits would this provide my condition?

- What does a reconstructed breast look and feel like?

- After surgery, will there be drains in my chest? Will they refer a nurse and wound specialist? (Ensure this referral is arranged BEFORE surgery regardless of whether you have drains in your chest!)

- Have them sign you up for a home health care aide prior to surgery.

- Are there any of the following available: financial aid/assistance to help me when I am off work? Social services? Health care services? Mental health services? Will the nurse navigator or hospital social worker help me obtain the same?

- Are there holistic options available for me to use before and/or after my surgery as I work toward recovery? Examples: yoga, meditation, chiropractic care, acupuncture, massage, reiki, etc.

- Will the breast surgeon send a sample of the tumor excised to be tested for cancer during the surgery?

- How many lymph modes are expected to be removed? Will sentinel only lymph nodes be removed? Is there a chance/determination that the cancer has already spread into the lymph nodes or elsewhere in the body? If so, would lymph nodes still need to be tested?

- What treatment is planned after surgery?

- If I have breast implants or stretchers placed in my breasts during surgery, what course of treatment will be followed? (i.e., home health aide, wound specialist, etc.)

- What if I am post-menopausal; what treatment will be recommended for me? How will I/my physician handle the numerous side-effects which WILL occur? (i.e., joint pain, bone density loss, hair loss, neuropathy in legs, imbalance, insomnia, migraines, etc.) Note: these are the standard side-effects experienced by women taking tamoxifen and aromatase inhibitors. It is up to each woman to decide for herself the quality of life she desires!

- Can I include holistic care in my treatment plan?

- If I am going to take the standard medicine (tamoxifen and aromatase inhibitors—estrogen blockers), why perform a mastectomy? Would a less invasive procedure such as a lumpectomy be a better choice?

- If you are only conducting one-sided lumpectomy, can the other breast be reconstructed to match? (This surgery is called an oncoplasty.)

- If you are conducting a mastectomy what is the level of scar tissue and neurological deficits I will experience?

- If you conduct a mastectomy, will you be able to conduct reconstruction of the breast on the same day?

- Is there a way to save my breast(s)?

- If my nipple(s) are involved and must be removed, what options do I have? Nipple reconstruction? Nipple removal? Nipple cleansing and reattachment?

- What sensations will I experience in my breast(s) after mastectomy or lumpectomy surgery?

- Would filling my breast(s) with body fat or tissue from other areas of my body jeopardize my ability to heal? Would cancer cells from other areas of my body (if present) jeopardize my health and make it more likely to contract cancer from another "infected" area?

- If you are using silicone implants, how will that affect my recovery or health?

- Will ovarian removal (hysterectomy) be conducted at the same time as my breast surgery? Would that cause recovery delays or place me at greater risk?

- Can we perform a transvaginal sonogram to determine whether my ovaries are actually involved or problematic prior to considering such a radical surgery as a hysterectomy or ovary removal merely as a preventive strike against *possible* **future** cancers if I am diagnosed with estrogen positive breast cancer? **If not, why not?** (Be careful as some surgeons will recommend ovary removal when there is no evidence to suggest that such a course of action is beneficial or warranted and is being suggested merely because your cancer was determined to be estrogen positive.)

- If ovary removal is recommended, is there an option to safeguard or harvest my eggs to allow future off-spring? (This will open an entire new line of questions and one you should discuss not only with your surgeon and oncologist but your gynecologist as well.)

- Why conduct preventive surgery when/if I'm placed on cancer medicines or chemotherapy?

- What level of breast shrinkage will be caused by radiation treatment? Will the plastic surgeon compensate for this variable during surgery? (Be sure to address this with the plastic surgeon.)

- Will a PET scan be conducted as well to determine if there is cancer anywhere else in my body?

- Will I be admitted into the hospital over night after my surgery? If not, why not?

Be mindful of "assembly line" mastectomy and lumpectomy surgeries where they send you home immediately. If you are not feeling well enough to be discharged, don't go home! If you are alone and have no one to take care of you or are a single mom, demand an overnight stay. It is your safety at risk! Yes, Medicaid and your insurance will pay for it if your surgeon requests it. If they send you home, and you do not feel it is appropriate, go to the emergency room and request to be admitted. Do not take risks with your life or your health!

- What plans are in place to address complications after surgery?

- What type of treatment and aftercare can I expect following my surgery?

- If my surgery is being performed in two or more stages/phases, please explain the risks in each stage/phase as well as the timing for each new stage/phase.

- Can/will radiation therapy be considered prior to surgery?

- When would I start radiation therapy?

- When would I be prescribed adjuvant therapy — tamoxifen or aromatase inhibitors?

- How does nutrition play a part in my cancer recovery? (Request a referral to the hospital nutritionist prior to and after surgery.)

- Are there any dietary supplements I should take to maintain or enhance my health?

- Will my reduction in weight affect my breast cancer or surgical recovery?

- What complications should I consider or keep an eye out for following surgery? (Discuss Sweet's syndrome.)

- Would it be best to await recovery of my breast surgery prior to ovarian surgery, if that is also recommended?

- What side effects will I experience in my arms or chest after surgery? Address lymphedema concerns.

- How can I prevent lymphedema? Can you schedule an appointment with a lymphedema specialist and/or physical therapist to discuss preventive measures?

- How will you detect any new cancer after my surgery?

- How often will I be evaluated with mammograms and sonograms after surgery?

- How will we manage my pain after surgery?

- Can you prescribe the pain medication and antibiotics which will be prescribed after surgery one or two days prior to surgery to ensure I have them available? If not, why not?

  The last thing you want to do is run to the pharmacy when you are in excruciating pain. Be sure to contact your pharmacy for possibilities of home delivery if your physician refuses to provide you with the medication ahead of time.

- Will I need to donate blood for my surgery?

- What will be the costs of my medication? (You can obtain this information from your pharmacist.)

- What side effects can I expect after surgery and from medication?

- If I will also undergo ovarian removal surgery or total hysterectomy, how long should I wait after breast surgery to perform it? Or will both operations be conducted at the same time? What is the risk factor given my age and current health for both scenarios?

- How will aging affect my breast conservation surgery?

- Will my surgical incision require plastic surgery to reduce scarring?

- What sleep positions should I avoid to prevent pain or injury to my chest?

- How can I avoid infection after surgery?

- How will I take care of my surgical wounds? Will a wound specialist be recommended? If not, why not?

- When can I anticipate a return to daily activities and/or work? What restrictions, if any, are anticipated?

- If I have thyroid cancer, will they remove my thyroid completely or partially? What are the pros/cons of each possibility?

- What type of treatment will be required if my thyroid is removed?

- What possible complications can occur during breast, thyroid or other surgery proposed?

- If ionized radiation or radiation seeds will be prescribed during and after surgery, what risks will these present to my health? (i.e., will I be at risk for leukemia? Is it best to avoid this treatment options?)

- How long will I have to remain on the medication prescribed? What side effects can I expect to encounter?

  There are always side effects! What you must consider is the quality of life you're willing to accept. Most of all, your decision should not be made from fear, guilt nor shame which sometimes is heaped on you by well-meaning physicians and loved ones.

- Will radiation be recommended after my surgery? If so, what type and duration? What are the risk factors?

- Is radiation recommended during/after surgery?

- What follow-up care will I be provided with from the breast surgeon and from the plastic surgeon?

- Will the breast/plastic surgeon follow-up with me to ensure I do not develop Sweet's syndrome? Will — can — a referral to a dermatologist be offered?

  Though Sweet's syndrome is a rare disorder, it is common when there is major trauma to an area — such as a lumpectomy and mastectomy. This disorder will prevent you from healing following surgery.

Note: Having a mastectomy is typically the standard choice of treatment for breast cancer over lumpectomies or no surgical treatment. However, there is NO GUARANTEE that you will be cancer free after a mastectomy nor that the cancer will not recur. Therefore, do not rush into a mastectomy out of fear. Consider all treatment options objectively. We've become a country accustomed to mastectomies being the treatment of choice even though several medical reports show there is no evidence to support that a mastectomy is more effective than a lumpectomy.

Regardless of your choice of treatment, there is always a possibility of recurrence despite the use of estrogen blockers such as tamoxifen, aromatase inhibitors or other medicines. It is up to you to assess the risk factors and determine how you wish to life your life. You can change the course of your treatment at any time; however, surgery is permanent.

I hope these questions provide you with ideas for your own. You can find more questions to ask in the American

Cancer Society's pamphlet on breast cancer and in other books discussing breast cancer treatment. Schedule an appointment with your nurse navigator to review them all. Record your session to enable you to have them for future reference. This will also allow you to share your Q&A session with your loved ones.

I found that my brain sometimes shut down during these discussions because of fear or feeling overwhelmed by my situation. The recordings were tremendously helpful and kept me from calling the doctor's office repeatedly for clarification and more questions. Note: it's OK to ask the same questions as often as you need to, especially if you do not understand the answers you are being provided.

Use the following pages to pose a few of your own questions and to jot down notes. I recommend putting the questions into your personal notebook alongside the answers.

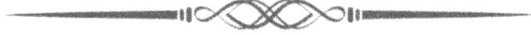

List your own questions/Notes:

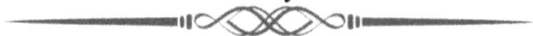

List your own questions/Notes:

CHAPTER 10

Things You SHOULD Know But AREN'T Told

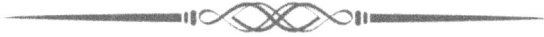

——————⟨◇⟩——————

When I first received my breast cancer diagnosis, I was voracious in my quest for information. So much so that the nurse navigator assigned to my case told me to stop reading and researching information. She joked that I was the equivalent of 10 patients combined when it came to the questions I asked and the information I craved.

I was, and still am, ferocious when it comes to learning about all aspects of cancer and how it relates to me, whether it's discovering aspects of my type of cancer, recommended treatment or possible alternatives and preventive measures. My friends joke that I'm getting a PhD in Cancer.

When one of my sisters was diagnosed with a lump on her left breast, she came to me for answers. I even had a few women I knew from various support groups ask me questions, even though they were diagnosed years before and had been on this journey much longer than I had.

This got me thinking about women and their choices, or at times lack of exploring them, which led me further into a deeper understanding of human nature.

I discovered there are two types of cancer patients. One type is proactive and researches this disease, including its corresponding issues and side effects. She (or he) asks questions and researches possibilities.

The other type of patient sits back and allow others to "deal with" the cancer for them. They're content following instructions and placing their treatment and any complications which arise in someone else's hands — in a way, giving up their responsibility to be a full participant in their treatment.

I understand the desire to stick your head in the sand like an ostrich and hide from cancer and the fear that death is eminent. I understand the need to believe and trust that your physician and other health care providers have all the answers and your best interests at heart.

There is no right or wrong in this. However, it's been proven that patients who take an active role in their health care have a better outcome.

Personally, I need to have some form of control in my life — even if it's as little as asking questions. I feel empowered when I research options and listen to my physician's advice, weighing the pros and cons of my situation and the effects surgery or medication will have on my life my body, and my mental health. Then, I make my decision for the type of treatment I will undergo.

It's not merely a matter of preference and personality. It's a matter of quality of life — your life!

You may discover it feels safer to ask questions, do research and learn all you can about this disease that has invaded your body and currently resides within you. Knowledge provides a sense of control. Knowing what's going on, what treatment options are available and what possible side effects you'll be faced with will help alleviate stress.

In my opinion, these two behaviors are akin to being prepared for the hurricane or waiting till it's upon you to board the windows and stock up on fresh water and food.

If you're reading this book, then you are looking for answers and taking an active role in your treatment. That's a wonderful thing! I commend you on your choice.

As you conduct your research, jot down any questions which pop into your mind; then ask your physician or nurse navigator. Don't worry that they won't listen or won't have time for you. If necessary, schedule a special appointment to ask your questions. If they won't address your questions or concerns, it may be time to look for a physician who will.

In case you didn't know, the nurse navigator is the nurse assigned to help answer questions and address your concerns. She'll help you schedule follow-up appointments and provide you with valuable information. She's one more resource at your disposal.

Unfortunately, some hospitals do not have a nurse navigator, or they may have limited resources available for you. Thus, do not rely solely on one person to advocate for you, have your *Cancer Tamer Posse* help.

Never forget, you are your own best advocate!

Take control of your life and live it to its fullest. Enlist your *Cancer Tamer Posse* to help you accomplish this goal.

Check out our *Resources* chapter for information on others who may be able to offer assistance, both financial and emotional. Work with your hospital's social worker or the VA (Veteran's Affairs) as they will be a valuable resource for you

Below are a few tidbits on information you should know but aren't told. They are issues I experienced as I went through my own breast cancer diagnosis, prepared for surgery and began treatment. I've also included some of my own musings and food for thought. Where possible, I've tried to separate the information into subjects or placed themes where they fit best;

though they are provided in random order within the categories provided.

Bathing

Though you won't need this bathing information until after surgery, I thought it would be important for you to know what you are facing and what will help you prepare.

- After surgery, you will have some restrictions on bathing for approximately seven to 10 days. You will be restricted from bathing your upper torso or getting your breast area wet. This, of course, is to prevent infection as you will have surgical bandages in place along with your compression bra. Do not remove these after surgery without your surgeon's consent — not even to change bras. You can use a damp wash cloth for your upper body and a bath/shower to clean your lower body. (Shower massagers with an eight-to twelve-foot length are a must have.)

- You will be able to wash your groin, butt and lower body after surgery. Having your partner bathe you is an intimate treat in itself. Not that it should lead to sex, nor would you be able to tolerate such activities shortly after surgery; however, having your partner bathe you will help to solidify your bond. You should get in the habit of doing this prior to surgery so it will not seem as awkward afterward. (Again, you can shower or bathe the lower portion of your body, ensuring you do not get your bandages wet.)

- If you have a home health aide, she can assist you with your shower or merely help prepare the shower or bath for you.

- After the bandages are removed, you will want to bathe with extra caution for your breasts, as they may be very sore and hypersensitive. If you are showering, I recommend you turn your back to the shower and allow the water to flow over your shoulder and onto your breasts. Direct pressure from the shower head will be painful. If you're bathing, use a plastic cup to pour the water against your upper shoulders and allow it to flow gently over your breasts. Do not scrub nor pick at the scabs. This could lead to infections or complications.

- When bathing, do not use perfumed soaps or scrubs on your breasts. Use natural washing gel or if using a bar of soap, be sure to get a lot of suds onto your hands and gently pass your hands over your breasts and under your arms where the lymph nodes were removed. I found using a washcloth or a sponge was too rough for the first two months after surgery. Be kind to your breasts, they've gone through a lot of trauma.

- One of the biggest obstacles with showering following your surgery will be washing your hair. Leaning forward will be difficult and cause tremendous pain, therefore, you won't be able to wash your hair in the sink. Washing it in the shower might lead to wetting your suture area and is not recommended. You could always try to sit in a chair and lean back into the sink or sit on the bathroom floor and lean back so your bandages don't get wet. The key factor here is not getting your bandages wet.

- Yes, you can visit a hair salon and have your hair washed and dried. Though convenient, dishing out the $30 or $40 for this service when you're trying to be frugal or don't have the money to spend can be stressful. That's why *Cancer Tamer* teamed up with several beauty salons to

provide you with a free or low-cost wash and rinse.
Please visit our website and register for your FREE membership to download the PDF for your FREE shampoo and blowout by Beauty Culture Academy in Staten Island or other beauty salons that have joined us. (If you know of a salon that would like to participate and offer a free or low-cost service to a woman after breast surgery, please let us know at info@CancerTamer.org.)

- On a side note, if you're planning to change the color of your hair, cover your gray or are ready for a new haircut, do so prior to surgery as you will not have the stamina for the time-consuming procedure, and you will want to avoid adding chemicals to your compromised system for the next few months.

Bras

What you wear after surgery is essential to your breast recovery. Below are a few tidbits to help you prepare for this aspect of treatment.

- After you're done with the compression bra which they'll place on you immediately after surgery — you'll awaken with it on — you'll need to wear bras which provide support but do not have an underwire. Remember, you'll have sutures on the outside of your breast(s) along the bra line. You'll also have many more sutures inside your body. You'll notice that old bras no longer fit you properly or sag — as will your clothes — a great excuse for a new wardrobe. You may also notice when removing your bra, you'll have a thin bloodline along the incision site. Typically, this may be caused by your bra sitting on your incision site. You may have not even felt the pressure from your bra as the area will be numb for months to come since many of the nerves were severed during surgery. Check your bra is fitting properly throughout the day. (As ever, speak with your physician if this or any other issues arise or if you have concerns.)

- When wearing bras, camisoles or anything else, avoid one which put pressure on your breasts or incision site. This will lead to pain, irritation and even possible bleeding. One of the most annoying experiences I had after surgery was finding a bra that fit correctly. Long and mid-line bras with larger adhesive strips at the bottom will be a great alternative for the next few months to ensure the bottom of the bra doesn't ride-up onto your suture line. (A mid-line bra is longer and comes to mid-torso.) As these bras are expensive, be sure to obtain a prescription from your doctor. Bras are considered durable medical equipment. This is also true of prosthetics necessary due to mastectomies.

- Mastectomy bras and compression bras can range from $40 to $70 or more. Medicaid and most insurance companies will pay for these bras if your physician prescribes them. (Yep, on a prescription pad.) You'll need a minimum of two bras — one to wear and one to wash. When you are recovering from surgery and unable to work, every cent counts. Do not be afraid nor ashamed to ask for what you're entitled to!

Breast Pain, Tweaks, Spasms and More

As you recover, you will notice that certain movements — or any movement for that matter — may cause pain, discomfort or spasms and tweaks to your breasts. This is normal. If you experience extreme pain or have concerns, always seek medical attention.

- Breasts are a part of your body that you can't ignore, like your arms or your legs. For women, they also hold center stage in our lives. Breasts contribute to how we feel about our bodies, ourselves and our femininity. Therefore, as you begin your cancer journey with your "new body," become acquainted with your "new breasts." Stimulate them by running your fingertips gently over them or massage them lightly once you've begun healing. This stimulation will awaken nerve endings and body memory, reminding your breasts of the sensations you experienced in the past. Most women fear touching themselves because of the taboos in our culture concerning masturbation. However, touching and reawakening the sensitivity in your breasts is not masturbation, it is a health requirement — a sensual health requirement!

Breast Self-Exam Following Surgery

Unfortunately, we're a society afraid of our own pleasure and of touching our own bodies. We need to start taking control of ourselves, our thoughts and the connections we make with our bodies and ourselves. Too many women are waiting for someone else to tell them there's something wrong — waiting for a doctor to perform a breast examine once a year — because they don't trust themselves or aren't comfortable exploring. Yet, what happens if you don't see the doctor for that yearly check-up? Who's checking your breasts then?

Never wait for someone else to ensure your health. You are the best, most reliable person to know your body and its changes. Examine your breasts monthly, if not weekly. This will allow you to detect any changes more readily. It will also help you in your sex life — but that's a discussion for another time.

Next time someone ask you if you're a feminist, tell them, "You're damn right I am. I reaffirm that freedom and power every time I perform my own breast examine."

Just as you wouldn't wait for someone to tell you to go to the bathroom, to change your clothes or to shower, don't wait for someone to tell you there's something wrong with your body — with your breasts. Check for yourself and check often!

Just because you've been diagnosed with breast cancer in one area doesn't mean you shouldn't continuously perform a full breast exam on both of your breasts as cancer can travel from one side of your chest to the other and elsewhere. They're your breasts, touch them often.

Dreams

Dreams are a powerful aspect of our lives. Understanding them is one way to improve your health, make better decisions and sleep better.

You may experience vivid or lucid dreams after your diagnosis. Like the famous psychiatrist, Carl Jung, I believe dreams are a pathway into your subconscious and unconscious mind. They hold and provide messages and truths you're not cognizant of during your waking hours. Discover the messages your dreams are trying to share. Sometimes, even nightmares will hold tremendous insight.

Personally, whenever I feel overwhelmed, I dream of zombies chasing me. When I feel like I need control in my life, I dream of being back in the military. You may even experience a fear of losing yourself and dreaming of death. These dreams are all perfectly normal occurrences.

One of the most vivid dreams I experienced shortly after being diagnosed was of a woman who died, yet only I remembered her. No one even realized she was dead — and worse yet, it seemed that they didn't even know she existed at all. I believe this dream reflected my sense of loss — of fear — that I was losing myself and who I once was.

If your dreams disturb you or you wish to make sense of them, discuss them with your physician and/or request an appointment with a psychologist or therapist to help you sort through them. There are psychologists and therapists who specialize in dream interpretation. Cancer Tamer Foundation hosts several workshops, even a few on how to interpret dreams.

Financial Resources

We all need a little help financially throughout our lives. Unless you're rich or have a year's worth of salary saved in the bank, you may find you'll need a little bit of finance assistance during your recovery. Below are a few resources to help you through the financial difficulties and challenges you may experience.

- Get your legal affairs in order. This isn't about whether you're going to die, it's about ensuring you are prepared for all eventualities. You need to have a health proxy, a last will and testament, a living will, and possibly a power of attorney. There are local organizations in your area which perform these services for free. There's a program in New York City called CAP (Cancer Advocacy Program). Check with your local congressperson's office or local district representative, as well as your hospital social worker. She will have valuable resources for you.
- Apply for Social Security Disability and Social Security Insurance within six months post-surgery if you're still off work. This is like flood insurance. The fact that you have cancer may push you to the front of the line and prompt them to review your case sooner. You will need to gather all your medical records for them to review. Thus again,

another reason to always obtain copies of your medical notes, tests, blood work, etc.

- If you are a veteran, regardless of when or how long you served, you may be entitled to VA benefits. Contact your local Department of Veterans Affairs (VA) office for further information.

- Contact the Department of Veterans Affairs if you're a veteran or the spouse of a veteran for assistance; they have organizations which may be able to help you financially if you fall behind on rent or need other assistance.

- Check out Rolling Thunder International. Their organization provides assistance to veterans and their loved ones.

- Stomp the Monster is a program that provides financial assistance to individuals with cancer. Check the internet for this and other programs.

- Become friendly with your hospital's social worker. He or she will be able to provide you with information about financial assistance or other programs. She will be a valuable resource and may also advocate on your behalf.

Holistic and Palliative Care
There are various treatment modalities available. Choose what's best for you. You can combine traditional western medicine with more holistic approaches. Many hospitals are now incorporating yoga, meditation and other forms of non-invasive treatment to their care options for cancer patients.

Holistic care is typically discussed after all other treatment options have been exhausted. It's like the last kid picked on a team. Yet, holistic care is now being seen as an important aspect of your health maintenance regime. It will help you prepare for surgery and help you keep a positive outlook on what lies ahead. The most important aspect of all is that it is non-invasive and has zero side effects, unlike most pain and cancer medications.

- Many individuals are not aware of palliative or holistic care. Several hospitals such as Mount Sinai and other well-known cancer institutions are turning toward holistic care (also known as palliative or supportive care) to aid in their cancer patient's recovery and help patients deal with the stressors and difficulties which lay ahead.

- Some forms of holistic care include: massage, relaxation and meditation, yoga, acupuncture, floating, low-impact exercise such as walking, reiki, energy work, sounds therapy and much more.

  Speak with your health care provider, nurse practitioner or hospital social worker as they can often refer you to the hospital's holistic care coordinator for further assistance. At the very least, get started with a little meditation and relaxation. The meditation tapes provided to me were a godsend and helped me through many nights where I lay in discomfort and was unable to sleep due to the pain following my surgery.

Home Health Care

If you're married, have children who can help or have family and friends to carry some of the weight during this challenging time, home health care won't be an issue. If you are single or alone and don't have a *Cancer Tamer Posse* to rely on, here are a few helpful tips.

- Request your surgeon authorize a visiting nurse. Typically, they won't do this unless you have drains put in; however, you can argue the fact that even without the drains you still need to have her come in to assess your situation and evaluate your need for a home health aide. If your surgeon, physicians or the nurse navigator will not assist you in this, contact your social worker. Don't take "no" for an answer. This is too important to your physical and mental health.

- It's not the doctor/surgeon's job to determine whether your insurance company will allow you or pay for a home health aide. The visiting nurse will evaluate your needs based on a discussion with you and an evaluation of your home and support system.

Insurance

Below are a few tidbits which relate to your health insurance and other insurance policies.

- Have your physician prescribe gauze pads size 4 by 4, and indicate you need to use 8 to 12 pads daily. (Enough for both breasts and changing the pads twice a day for 30 days at a time.) Your physician may give you a few at the office; however, it won't last you long and purchasing a box of 25 pads at the local pharmacy will cost you approximately $5.25 per box. You'll go through a box in less than a week, and though $5.25 seems like a nominal fee, it'll quickly grow to $50 a month or more for several months. Don't forget you'll have many more expenses to cover as you recover that your insurance may not cover, including vitamins, zinc and Xeroform to help you heal.

- Sometimes your insurance company will deny a vitamin or prescription because it's in capsule form; however, they'll approve it if it's in tablet form. Or they'll want the generic formula of the vitamin. Though it seems foolish of them to approve one form and not the other, it's part of their internal bureaucracy. Don't try fighting it, it'll drive you nuts or make you depressed — I'm speaking from experience on this — just have your doctor prescribe the medicine again based on the insurance company's specifications.

- It is not your physician's responsibility to decide what your insurance will or will not pay for. Ask them to prescribe everything you need and then you or your advocate — a member of your *Cancer Tamer Posse* — can address any denials.

   Though physicians are used to dealing with various insurance companies, I found that exceptions can be made. This includes a home health aide which most plans, including Medicaid and Medicare, **will** cover if requested by your physician or a medical provider. Your social worker can also put in the request.

- Check with your credit card companies and your home insurance policy; sometimes there is a provision where they will pay your minimum payment if you are unable to work. It may require a letter from your physician.

Never take "no" for an answer until you have considered and exhausted all the possibilities.

Lymphedema
Lymphedema is a condition which may arise because your lymph nodes were removed. This condition typically occurs on

the arm where your lymph nodes were removed. Lymphedema presents as an abnormal swelling of your arm(s) and can lead to circulation and extreme health issues. Once you have lymphedema, you'll have it for life; thus, do all you can to prevent it.

- To help prevent and avoid lymphedema, do not allow your blood nor blood pressure to be taken from the arm where your lymph nodes were removed — **ever!** If lymph nodes were removed from under both your arms, have your blood pressure and blood taken from your thigh or ankle as the tourniquet used when drawing blood causes too much pressure to your arm and will cause lymphedema. Avoid it at all costs.

- When traveling in an airplane, ensure to wear a compression sleeve on the arm(s) where the lymph nodes were removed. Speak to your doctor about this and have them prescribe a compression sleeve, gauntlet and/or glove. Your insurance should cover it with a physician's prescription.

- To help prevent lymphedema during the hot summer months, place a cold pack under your armpits. Also, limit your time in saunas and hot tubs as extreme changes in body temperature can lead to lymphedema.

- Report any infections or injuries to your arms immediately; this includes infections from having your cuticles removed at the nail salon. (Of course, it is obvious that you should ensure the salon uses only sterilized cuticle removers when doing your nails.)

- Consult a certified lymphedema therapist for a lymphatic drainage massage once a month or more regularly as prescribed by your physician. Yes, most insurance companies pay for this treatment; however, you may have to fight for it — this is one of those fights worth having.

Mental and Physical Health

Though mental and physical health greatly impacts our quality of life, many of us overlook it. Below are a few aspects to keep in mind as the months and years ahead go by.

- It's almost impossible to relax and hyperventilate at the same time; however, as a cancer patient, you'll feel like this happens to you often, especially after first being diagnosed. Be sure to make time for yourself to relax and de-stress. Immerse yourself in your favorite hobby for a few hours a week. Go for a walk — no cell phones. Listen to music that you love to sing along with. Take a drive. Forget about cancer for a while. It'll be there waiting for you when you return stronger and more fortified than ever to *tame your cancer*.

- Join a support group for cancer patients in your age group and for your specific cancer diagnosis. If the first group meeting you attend doesn't work for you, that's okay, seek another. Support groups are like everything else in life, you must find the correct fit for it to be most effective.

- Communicate your feelings with others. I know I've said this before; however, it bears repeating, if you don't feel comfortable discussing your cancer diagnosis with someone or their platitudes annoy you, remind them — respectfully of course — that though you realize they mean well, you would prefer they not continue their comments.

This includes well-meaning friends, family and strangers who will share their stories, beliefs and more.

During my search for an apartment, the real estate woman decided to explain to me how God would cure my cancer if I only believed more. This was annoying as hell since she didn't know my spiritual beliefs and began to dictate how I should "speak" about my cancer. All in the space of 20 minutes of meeting me.

Keep in mind they mean well; however, they can be intrusive and offensive. Thus, communicate your preferences and your needs for boundaries in a respectful and firm manner whenever necessary.

Nutrition

Nutrition is always on the menu, and something you must consider from now on. Living healthy is a choice to make every day. Your life depends on it. The old adage, "your body is your temple," is something to keep at the forefront of your mind. If you return to old unhealthy habits after surgery, you may set yourself up for unhealthy consequences as well as recurrence. Let this situation be your wake-up call for better health.

- Cancer thrives on sugar. When making smoothies with lots of fruit, ensure to balance it out with some green vegetables. Though having a sugar-free diet may be out of your present future, you can begin cutting back on sugar slowly. Ironically, you will discover how much more energy you have without it. Keep in mind you do not want to use artificial sugar substitutes as those may cause their own problems, and some have been linked with cancer. Yes, it can be a pain in the butt to eat healthy and avoid sugar and soy if you've been diagnosed with estrogen positive breast cancer as soy is in almost everything we eat. However, little by little, you can create the nutritional balance your body needs.

- Be conscious of the foods you purchase. Yes, this means reading the ingredients. If your breast cancer is estrogen positive, doing so is essential. You will be shocked at all the food products which contain estrogen. These include, but aren't limited to, nutritional bars and chips. Yep, many nutritional bars use soy as an "adhesive" for their foods. Chocolate, even pure or natural/organic chocolate may contain soy. I can hear you groaning now over this fact, however, there are some companies who do not use soy in their chocolate. Research. **You must be vigilant and read the labels. Your health depends on it!**

  I've found over 90 percent of all the candies I love have soy lecithin in it, as do many ice creams. And believe it or not, some organic trail mixes contain soy as well. Soy seems to be in almost everything. Do I need to mention soy sauce, soy milk and tofu? If you're breast cancer is ER positive, you must limit the soy intake in your diet. Just because you're choosing to take aromatase inhibitors doesn't mean that the soy you're putting into your body through your diet will be "blocked" by your medicine. Speak with your nutritionist and oncologist.

  Cancer Tamer will be providing a few workshops on nutrition as we work with our Medical Advisory Board; thus, keep an eye out for updates on our website. **www.CancerTamer.org.**

- It's perfectly acceptable and even preferable if you begin experimenting with making your own meals. If you're not a cook, keep things simple. If you enjoy cooking or want to learn, invest in a few cookbooks. Consider eating gluten free; alternate starchy pastas, which will turn to sugar, for vegetable pasta such as zucchini, squash, spinach, etc.

Consider adding vegetables and fruits into your diet. Review the chapter on **Creative Nutrition** for some delicious recipes. Search for a nutritionist that will help you with your quest to eat healthier. Remember you can change any recipe to your individual tastes.

- Check into meal delivery. Some insurance programs will allow you to have home delivered meals if you have a home health aide assigned to you for over 28 to30 hours a week. Choose healthy meals!

You don't have to become a *crazy health freak*, just be conscientious of what you put into your body. In the end, eating healthy is a choice you make every time you eat or drink.

Second Opinions

Just as you ask your girlfriends what they think about what you're wearing, your new shoes or a potential boyfriend, a second opinion regarding your surgery and treatment is not something you want to pass-up.

- Take the time to obtain a second or even a third opinion about your surgical options. Don't rush into surgical options merely out of fear or confusion. Unless your condition is so dire that surgery is imperative immediately, you have a few weeks' — even months' — time in which you can solicit opinions from other medical professionals. As I've mentioned several times, the unvarnished and bitter truth is that once you have surgery, no other surgeon will touch you, especially if something has gone wrong! No one wants to step in somebody else's crap. This happened to me. It is one of the reasons I stress this throughout the book as I do not want you to have to experience the insanity that comes with such a situation.

- When speaking with a surgeon, you'll want to ask them about aftercare. What will they do for you? What treatments they recommend? If your physician is not available and complications arise, are there other surgeons you can seek advice from in their practice or with an affiliate or colleague? Who are those individuals? (Contact them and have a discussion with them **prior** to surgery.)

- If you're on Medicaid/Medicare or a federal program, don't feel like you should accept what's given to you. You are entitled to choose your level and type of care. You may be limited in the hospitals or physicians who will accept your coverage. However, I've met and know so many wonderful physicians and surgeons who take low income health insurance. Shop around. Talk to prior patients.

- Most physicians are now online; check them out on the internet. Don't be fooled into believing that they're great just because they are the head of their department or because they have magazine covers stating they've been voted as one of the "Top 100 in Your State."

- The best judge and the best resource of information are current and prior patients. You can easily discover these individuals in the doctor's waiting room. Patients love to talk about their surgery. Share your concerns and ask them about their level of care and how any complications were handled. Did the physician act on the patient's concerns? Were they referred to other providers? Did that physician/plastic surgeon merely say, "*This is normal,*" when things were not progressing? If so run from that physician!

Sexuality

You are a sensual human being. Though sex may be the furthest thing from your mind at the moment, it won't be as the months and years progress. Speak with your partner and your physician(s) about how your condition, the surgery, treatment and the medications prescribed will affect your sex life. We will discuss sex and intimacy in more detail in book two of the series, *Breast Cancer: From Surgery thru Treatment.*

Unfortunately, we are a society that is afraid of our own pleasure, of touching our bodies. This stigma was perpetuated by Richard von Krafft-Ebing in 1886 in his book, *Psychopathia Sexualis* which stated that lust murderers began their slip into madness through masturbation. For over a century after his book, society still has a negative reaction toward anything sexual. We need to start taking control of ourselves, our thoughts, our connections and our bodies.

Don't wait for a physician to tell you something is wrong with your body, perform your own breast exam and when in doubt, have your doctor check it out.

Did you know that over 70 percent of all breast cancers are detected by the woman herself?

Performing your own breast exam will also allow you to become familiar with your breasts, especially after surgery. Just as you wouldn't wait for someone to tell you when to go to the bathroom or change your clothes, don't wait nor depend on others to tell you there's something wrong with your breasts. Check for yourself and check often! And as a bonus, let your lover or spouse perform the breast exam for you. It could just lead to a lot more fun.

Warning: If you are BRCA1 or BRCA2 positive and/or estrogen positive, there may be a "push" from your physicians to have your ovaries removed as well. Ovarian removal or a full hysterectomy is a radical approach! Before considering such a radical course of action, it's imperative to have a second or third opinion.

Become an active participant in your treatment plan. Listen to the options available and discuss them with family, your spouse, your friends, even other physicians. You also want to consider all aspects of your health and the possibility of complications to your physical, emotional and sexual well-being.

Yes, you do need to consider your sexual health. Do you want to continue being a sexual human being after surgery and enjoy sex to its fullest potential, or are you willing to compromise your sexual future? Having a full hysterectomy comes with its own set of complications, including possible sexual dysfunctions such as pain during intercourse and anorgasmia (inability to be orgasmic). Thus, consider your options closely.

One of the reasons the breast surgeon will immediately want to remove your ovaries is because they produce estrogen, and if your breast cancer is estrogen positive, this will be an issue. However, don't overlook the fact that your body needs estrogen to function, and some studies show it may also aide in preventing heart attacks. If you decide to follow the adjuvant chemotherapy protocol of tamoxifen and aromatase inhibitors, these drugs will reduce your body's ability to absorb and produce estrogen.

This is a dialogue you must have with your physician in great length to determine what is best for you medically, as well as for the quality of life you wish to have.

Sleep

Sleep can be elusive at times. Speak with your physician if you find it difficult falling asleep, staying asleep or have insomnia. Sometimes instituting "quiet time" an hour prior to your bed time will be helpful. Below are a few tidbits to consider.

- You may find it difficult to sleep after being diagnosed with cancer. This is normal. If it becomes a major nuisance, speak with your physician. Building in quiet time to prepare for bed will be very helpful. For instance, a half-hour to an hour before your typical bedtime, turn off the television, get off the computer and disconnect for mental stimulus. Drink some herbal tea made for sleep, read a book, take a bubble bath, etc. Whatever helps you to unwind. Getting at least seven to eight hours of sleep will help you not only feel more energized but help speed up your healing process.

- If you suffer from insomnia, try taking daily naps for 15 to 30 minutes. It won't interfere with your nightly sleep. You may find these naps give you the added boost you need to keep going during the day. Stay away from energy drinks! They're typically full of sugar and steroids — two things cancer thrives on.

- After surgery, it'll be difficult to sit up, lay on your stomach or even your sides (both of which put pressure on your chest) for at least three to six months due to your sutures and your breasts readjusting and reshaping. What I found helpful was using pillows to prop myself up or keep me from rolling over. If you have a partner or someone sleeping in your bed, you can have them stay close so if you do turn in your sleep, you'll bump up against them and adjust yourself. Be careful with small children or a partner who flays around a lot lying beside you; accidental bumps against your chest can be painful.

Supplements and Vitamins

Always discuss all medications, vitamins and supplements with your oncologist and medical physicians.

- Zinc is a supplement you'll need to help in your healing and recovery. Discuss its use with your physician. Ask them to provide you with a prescription, and see if your insurance will cover it. As I mentioned before, though it's a miniscule amount to purchase this supplement, when you add up all your other expenses, you may discover you're spending $100 to $200 monthly on supplements and supplies alone. This doesn't include the $100s you may spend on cancer medications.

- Be careful when taking over-the-counter supplements while undergoing chemotherapy or radiation as some vitamins and supplements will interfere with the chemo uptake and cause difficulties.

- Peppermint tea is great for reducing and eliminate nausea.

- Whenever possible, eat more fruits and vegetables as getting nutrients and vitamins straight from the source is the best option. Try juicing as an alternative to soft drinks or energy drinks which are full of sugar and feed your cancer.

- Be sure to have your physician prescribe a calcium supplement with vitamin D to enable your body to absorb it. This will help you avoid the onset of osteoporosis which **will** occur due to the radiation treatments and the aromatase inhibitors or tamoxifen medication prescribed. It's not a matter of **IF** it'll occur, but **WHEN** it'll occur if you are taking cancer medications. Help yourself stay healthier longer.

Surgery

As discussed throughout this book, ensure to conduct your research and ask questions prior to surgery. Below are a few more tidbits you may find useful. I apologize if I sound like a mother hen; however, I've been through the good and the very bad of surgery and treatment. I hope you this book helps you to avoid the same.

- What is the surgery being proposed? Is there a less invasive procedure possible? What are the risk factors? Given your age, other medical conditions, and/or healing difficulties (if any), is this the best surgical option for you? What is your expected recover time?

- What's the anticipated outcome of the surgery? How much breast area will be affected? What is the level of intensity of the surgery being performed? Would it be better to have a simpler surgery? How will they care for you after the surgery?

- Don't have extensive surgery if you don't have to. Do not allow fear to dictate your treatment choices. Review the chapter on *Preparing for Surgery* for more information.

- Though many aspects of cancer are scary, you are bright and intelligent, and if they explain it to you in terms you understand, you'll be able to grasp it easily. Don't allow yourself to be driven by fear or be bullied into a specific surgery or treatment plan. You're a smart adult; weigh your options.

Sweet's Syndrome

I was diagnosed with a rare auto-immune disorder called Sweet's syndrome. Yep, sweets like candy. This is where your body has experienced trauma in a specific area and your immune system goes on hyperdrive and sees everything as an invasion, including healthy and healing tissue.

Though it's said to be a rare immune disorder, given my preliminary research, talking to women and reviewing pictures of breast cancer patients online (something I do not recommend as it's terrifying to see all the complications women with breast cancer can experience), I believe Sweet's syndrome is very prevalent in breast cancer patients and goes undiagnosed because the surgeons/plastic surgeons and their staff do not look for it, aren't aware of it, or as my dermatologist stated, surgeons don't look outside the box and are too egotistical to ask for help.

It was a shock to hear my plastic surgeon declare that after ten plus years of surgical practice, he'd learned something new, when I shared my dermatologist's findings with him. I was flabbergasted as I knew I couldn't have been the only patient in over 10 years that developed this auto-immune disorder; that means many other women suffered from this condition because he never researched what was happening to them. His idea of dealing with my complications was merely stating, "It's normal." He waited eight weeks before stating that I needed emergency surgery to correct the complications to my condition.

If Sweet's syndrome goes untreated, you may undergo several surgeries with the same undesired results — suture dehiscing, infections, and further complications. Your mental health will also suffer as you are forced to watch your breasts' deterioration — and possible skin rotting — daily as you look in the mirror, shower, put on your bra.

Breasts are an integral part of your body, directly related to a woman's self-image and identity. Do not allow anyone to tell you otherwise. Learn about this auto-immune disorder to prevent its complications and scarring should you develop it.

This condition is so invasive and causes so much damage to your breasts and mental health that I felt compelled to add it to this book. It's also why I believe any woman undergoing breast surgery should also be under the care of a dermatologist and be evaluated for any healing issues which arise immediately. **Immediately — as in two weeks following surgery — not longer!**

If you are not healing within two weeks of surgery and your stitches start to dehisce (let go), speak to your surgeon about a referral to a dermatologist. As dermatologists are extremely busy, have your surgeon or primary physician call in a favor so you can be seen immediately (within the week). I also recommend you schedule your appointment to be seen by the dermatologist prior to your surgery as they are always booked and hard to get into see.

The treatment for Sweet's syndrome is fairly simple and consists of steroid injections into the infected site. **If left untreated, you will not heal.** Worse yet, you will develop tremendous scars on your breasts and your nipples may be in jeopardy.

As with any treatment, speak to your physician. Address concerns. Most of all do research. You are your own best advocate.

To learn more about Sweet's syndrome, please review our website for our television show on this topic. There are also a few pictures on the webpage of a breast with Sweet's syndrome that may be a little upsetting; however, they show the progression of this disorder. **http://cancertamer.org/list-of-shows/sweet-syndrome**.

A million thanks to Dr. Jacob Levitt, dermatologist, our guest on this segment of Cancer Tamer Television Talk Show and the physician who diagnosed my condition and cured it — and most important of all, saved what was left of my breasts.

Tests

Some tests will be simple procedures, others may cause you a bit of anxiety. Below are a few tidbits to help you through it.

- When having an MRIs or any examinations performed which have a magnetic component to them, speak with your physician about piercings and even permanent eye makeup. Some permanent eye makeup contains metal flecks which will interfere with MRI machines and cause you pain and discomfort; it may also cause your eyelids to swell. Discuss these possibilities with your physician and the MRI technician.

- One great benefit to genetic testing is the fact that you'll have justification for your insurance company to be monitored closely and have tests performed more often. For instance, you have the option of having an MRI scan performed every six or 12 months, or having your colon checked every two years versus every five years. Be sure to keep track of all follow-up appointments and their frequency. Establish a baseline of your health, blood, tumor marker tests, vitamin deficiencies, etc., and chart your progress based on present and past results. The downside to genetic testing is the fear and anxiety it can provoke if you test positive in any area/gene. All too often women will opt for pre-emptive mastectomies and full hysterectomies when monitoring or minimal surgery would be best.

- I know I've stated this in other areas of this book; however, it bears repeating — just because your genetic test came back positive for the BRCA1 or BRCA2 gene (or any other gene related to cancer) **does not** signify you'll develop cancer. It merely indicates you're at higher risks **IF** you don't take care of yourself. If you don't provide your body with good nutrition, adequate sleep, exercise and mental balance, or if other environmental factors are present, you MAY develop cancer.

- I caution you about jumping off the "fear cliff" and into surgery without weighing all the possible complications. Check out Dr. Bruce Lipton's fabulous lecture on the epigenetics of life. I'd also recommend his book, *The Biology of Belief.* Though you may find the first two chapters a little hard to follow if you're not familiar with biology, the rest of the book is easy to absorb and a thrill to read. Dr. Lipton helps you discover how chronic conditions such as cancer can develop and how you can *tame your cancer* by simply changing your behaviors and eating patterns.

- Ask your physician to conduct a bone density test to establish a baseline for yourself and assess any osteoporosis or osteopenia which may be present. This test should be performed yearly. It will help you determine the effects — damage — of the medications you're taking, such as tamoxifen and aromatase inhibitors, on your skeletal system. This will also help them determine treatment options to help you keep your bones healthy and prevent future complications such as broken bones and hips.

Treatment

Here are a few treatment options and situations you should be aware of. As ever, consult your medical provider(s) if you experience any of these situations to determine the best course of treatment for your condition. As mentioned previously, these recommendations are from my personal experience and what worked best in my situation and are not intended to be provided as medical advice.

- Keep a journal of all your appointments. Notate whom you're visiting and why, as well as the outcome of the visit and what treatment was provided. Also make note of any follow-up care required. This will be very important as time progresses. You will undergo many treatments, appointments, consultations, etc. over the course of your treatment and the years to come. It will be difficult to keep track of it all as the months and years go by. If you choose the medical options to undergo chemo or radiation therapy, these treatments will affect your memory. Having this information will not only be helpful to you, it will also help your spouse or *Cancer Tamer Posse* as well as. It'll also come in handy for any further insurance or legal situations you may encounter.

- Sweet's syndrome is a rare and often undiagnosed auto-immune disorder which will prevent or delay your body's ability to heal. I've spoken of it several times. Please check into it if you're not healing properly following surgery. Sweet's syndrome is but one condition which will keep you from healing. Check with an infection disease physician and/or dermatologist for other possibilities.

- It's sad to say, however we — women — have become socially conditioned to mutilate ourselves out of fear. I know that's harsh to say, yet it's true. Too many women have chosen a mastectomy out of fear when in some cases a lumpectomy or no surgery at all may be just as effective or the better option, according to medical research. Don't let fear control you! Before agreeing to extensive surgery, get those second and third medical opinions.

- Speak with your physician about the use of Xeroform wound care gauze pads. They are specially treated gauze pads which help promote healing. Nope, your surgeon will not immediately prescribe these. They're expensive. However, if they are prescribed, your insurance company should pay for them. They are billed under "durable medical equipment" even though you toss them out after one use. You may have to "fight" with your insurance carrier for them to be accepted; however, it's well worth it as it promotes healing and reduces scaring.

Typically, Xeroform gauze pads will cost you approximately $45 to $65 for a box of 50 pads. You'll use that many or more in a month. Ask for the 5-by-9 pads. You can then cut the 5 by 9s in half and use   half on each breast. Don't purchase the 4 by 4s; they're too small if you've had breast reconstruction, and you'll merely need to use two on each breast. Your physician needs to prescribe these; yep, on a prescription form! Have them prescribe the use of four a day for 30 days. You can always refill the prescription.

Note: If your insurance company denies you, speak with your insurance nurse representative. Have her get this approved on your behalf. You should connect with her immediately after/prior to surgery so she's aware of your needs. She'll also be a major asset to your ***Cancer Tamer Posse.).***

- Some women experience vaginal and fungal infections (otherwise known as yeast infections) due to antibiotics. Speak to your physician/surgeon and ask them to prescribe DeFlucan or another similar medicine to help prevent a yeast infection at this delicate time. The last thing you want to experience is pain in your vaginal area when you're experiencing pain in your breasts. You may not even notice the vaginal discomfort right away as your body is focused on the pain in your breast(s).
If prescribed, you'll want to take the DiFlucan as soon as you start the antibiotics. Don't wait until your discomfort

turns painful; you'll be in enough discomfort from the breast surgery. If you're prone to yeast infections, speak with your surgeon about this. (Note: over-the-counter products such as Monostat may not work as effectively.) As ever, speak with your physician about any medications needed and their potential side effects.

- Drinking cranberry juice and eating yogurt may help prevent and/or alleviate the side effects of yeast infections. For those with lactose intolerance or who don't wish to drink milk because of all the steroids and other chemicals fed to cows and transferred to the milk, Silk has a new yogurt made of almond milk which is delicious and comes in various flavors. There are also other non-dairy products on the market.

- Demand, if necessary, that they send someone to help you with wound care. Though it may seem like a no-brainer to take off gauze pads and replace them with new sterile ones (and they teach you at the hospital how to empty your drains), you'll want to have someone trained in your home to ensure you're doing the procedure correctly. The wound specialist can also keep an eye on you to ensure your wounds and incision site are healing properly and provide early detection of any medical concerns.

- If you're not healing, be sure to visit your doctor weekly, not monthly as they may recommend. Take photos of your breasts daily to note your condition and **demand** to be seen. Sometimes these photos will help them better understand your condition. Also, request an appointment with an infectious disease specialist and/or dermatologist who will be able to diagnose any complications you're experiencing faster than your typical breast and plastic surgeon. My plastic surgeon waited over 12 weeks before he addressed my wound care despite my repeated concerns and weekly visits. It wasn't until I threatened a lawsuit that his partner referred me to a dermatologist to assess my condition for possible immune disorders, and at that point, my condition was treated properly.

Note: We did not address the use of chemotherapy prior to treatment in this book as it is being covered in my second book in this series, ***Breast Cancer: From Surgery thru Treatment.*** Please reference that book for ideas and tidbits on how to deal with the effects of chemotherapy and radiation therapy as well as the side effects associated with them pre/post-surgery.

This is your health. Be your own best advocate!

Tidbits

Below are a few additional tidbits I thought you should know that didn't fall easily within the other categories provided. Though, I know there are many more tidbits that I won't be able to cover in this book, I hope those I have will get you started on your journey and provide you with a springboard to use for your own research. Feel free to share your own tidbits with us on our website.

- Purchase an old-fashioned washboard to wash your bras after surgery. This will allow you to remove some of the stains caused by the Xeroform gauze pads and/or the bits of dried blood your washing machine may not get this clean. You can purchase a washboard online.

- You may find it difficult to sit up or lay down after surgery. Use pillows to prop yourself up and to keep you from rolling over onto your side or stomach. If you're cuddling up with your sweetheart, find a position that's most comfortable for you. You may need to switch sides on the bed due to your lymph nodes being removed on a particular side. That's okay, change is good. If snuggling is uncomfortable, holding hands in bed; tangling your feet is always a fun and intimate way to connect.

- Just because you've been diagnosed with breast cancer in one area, doesn't mean you shouldn't continuously perform a full breast exam on yourself on both breasts as cancer can travel from one side of your chest to the other and elsewhere.

- You may not be able to lift an 8-ounce bottle/glass of water after surgery. Place a small plastic bottle with a bendy straw by your bed for when you get thirsty in the middle of the night. Another trick to use is to place your medicines (pain pills and antibiotics) in a small bowl by the water on your nightstand. This will make it easier for you to take and recall if you've already taken the dosage for that timeframe. (Be careful using this option if you have small children or pets at home.)

- I recommend you join a support group for cancer patients, one with your specific diagnosis; i.e., breast cancer, ovarian cancer, etc. They are a great resource. It's always comforting to be with others who understand the challenges you are facing. That said, support groups are like shoes; you need to find the one that fits best for you. There are various groups available, even ones which differentiate by age as some patients will feel more comfortable with members their own age. There are online support groups as well.

- As you recover from surgery, you will notice that certain movements (or any movement for that matter) may cause pain, discomfort, spasms or tweaks in your breasts. This is normal. I often joked that "crazy coyotes" were using plungers to pull out my breasts, trying to make them bigger once more after my surgery; or that the pain and discomfort were my breast's way of saying it was "pissed." To alleviate the discomfort, I used my lymphedema pillow or my hands to hold my breasts. I also massaged them lightly. Don't be afraid to touch your breasts — after all, it's your body!

- Some friends and family members will want to know intimate details of your surgery and how treatment is progressing, including how your sutures and scars look. They may even insist on a visual. It's perfectly acceptable for you to set limits and explain that beyond a certain point, or as your healing progresses, you're uncomfortable discussing certain aspects of your treatment or showing your scars. It's up to you how much you share and with whom. You can take photos to show them and avoid the more personal aspect of exposing your actual breasts to them.

- Here is a list of a few items you will need which are covered by most insurance. In some instances, you will need genetic or scientific formula for the vitamins. Though they're only a few dollars each, those dollars will quickly add up to $25, $50, even $100 or more a month. Whenever possible, have your insurance pay for them. These are: gauze pads, Xeroform, vitamins B12, B6, C, D and calcium. Some insurance will also cover zinc.

- Your breasts will look different after surgery and throughout the healing process. I found it helpful to take photographs of my breasts daily as it provided documentation for my plastic surgeon when my condition worsened, and I developed complications. This may be something that works for you as well. I took the photos on my smartphone. These photos also came in handy when I didn't feel comfortable displaying my breasts and healing progress to physicians or loved ones/partner. It's a great way to document your progress.

- Be sure to obtain your medical notes and any tests which are performed immediately; at a minimum monthly. This will ensure you have copies you'll need handy for other physicians, as well as SSI/SSD and other financial organizations. (You may be surprised to learn information about treatment options your physician did not share.)

- Contact the Cancer Tamer Foundation for lymphedema pillows to help alleviate pain after surgery.

- Create a video for yourself and loved ones which conveys words of wisdom and your wishes for their future. This video will also serve as a time capsule of sorts for you in the future where you can provide your thoughts and encouragement for yourself. Review it often, especially when you find yourself struggling to go on. Contact Cancer Tamer Foundation to schedule a time to record your **"Here and Now"** video.

<u>Thoughts and Musings</u>

Below are a few thoughts and musings I've had as the months went by. Feel free to jot down your own in your journal book. You're also welcomed to share them with me or post them on our website's blog section for discussion.

- False platitudes are annoying as hell. Be cognizant of what annoys you and have an in-depth conversation with others to help avoid future problems and resentments.

- When you feel your life is getting off course, merely "redirect" yourself in the direction you want to go. It's like fine tuning a piano, you must do it often to maintain the perfect pitch. You're going through tremendous emotional turmoil at the moment. Life is and will continue to be off kilter for a little while. That's OK; adjust when and however you feel is appropriate for you.

- As Mike Dooley says, "Thoughts become things." What you believe becomes your reality. Therefore, keep faith in yourself and your future throughout these challenging times. Find ways to make yourself feel joy. Get a bracelet that says, "Choose." Or write the word on your arm daily to remind yourself that life and how you live it **IS** your choice. Determine for yourself what you want to experience, and create it in your life. This is the "post-cancer surgery you," and she's amazing!

- Love yourself. Be proud of yourself. If not now, when?

- Angels come from all walks of life and at the weirdest moments. It's in their actions, their words, their presence that we'll have a moment of clarity, of hope, of peace. Recognize these moments. Cherish them. They'll always appear when you need them most.

- Remind yourself of this truth: you will never lose the battle against cancer; though one day you will die just as everyone else will. Therefore, choose to live every day to the fullest. That's the real way to "battle" cancer.

- Fear can make you procrastinate. Make you hide from the truth. Make you avoid "knowing." However, you're stronger than whatever life throws your way. You can handle it — you always have.   .

- It's alright to become an ostrich and hide your head in the sand for a day or so. I've done so myself several times after my diagnosis — choosing to stay in bed and lock out the world. But after a day or two of bingeing on TV shows or other habits that weren't productive, I still had to face the truth of my diagnosis and make hard decisions which affected my health and my future. Thus, feel free to take a day or two to be an ostrich, then embrace the powerful woman you hold within and face life. Create your own path.

- Listen to your inner voice — always. I recall vividly sitting in my oncologist's office as she recommended chemotherapy, and I swear I heard my soul screaming, "Please don't poison me. I'll be good. I'll be good!"

    It is perfectly acceptable to refuse chemotherapy and/or radiation treatments. Thousands of patients do. It is your right to choose or deny the treatment options presented to you. Sometimes, treatment will not provide you with improved odds or have limited or minimal benefits; this is when you must weigh the risks and the benefits.

    Always speak with your physician(s) and obtain second and third opinions to determine the best course of treatment for you if you have any concerns or doubts, or just to assure yourself the course of treatment recommended is the best for you.

    Personally, I sought my second and third oncology opinions at different hospitals to ensure objectivity.

Ultimately the choice to have or deny treatment is yours!

- It's perfectly normal and appropriate to mourn the loss of your breasts or hair loss. Speaking with a therapist, the hospital oncology social worker or a trusted friend about this issue can help.

- Find ways to keep your attitude positive and playful. Personally, I use humor to help me cope, especially when I'm feeling scared or not at my "superwoman" strength. One of the jokes I often use is, "breast cancer is good for your posture." This is because leaning forward and not sitting up straight will cause discomfort. Okay, I realize that joke may be a little lame, but it makes me smile every time. And it makes me laugh to see other's reactions when I say it. Their expressions are priceless.

- I've always loved Tim McGraw's song, "Live Like You Were Dying." Now, I interpret and internalize the lyrics on an entirely different level. Consider for a moment what it would be like to live each day to the fullest. To have every moment in your life be special, meaningful, precious — yeah, even the difficult ones. Amazing thought, isn't it?

- No one wants to talk about death. Every time I brought up the topic, my friends and medical staff avoided it or dismissed the topic altogether. That is their hang-up not mine. Talk about death with yourself, with your support group, or with a trusted friend who will let you share your thoughts and fears. This does not mean you're suicidal. It merely demonstrates that you're being realistic and addressing the elephant in the room — the possibility of your death — your mortality. Doing so is actually quite healthy.

I remember speaking to one of the counselors that I was seeing about my belief that I would die on the operating table. He chided me for "thinking negatively." Yet, I wasn't being negative, I was simply stating a fear I had as everyone in my family who had been diagnosed with cancer had died.

Though people mean well, you do need to find someone, a support group or a trained professional, who can address all your concerns, including death. The way I look at it is simple; it all comes down to one question: "When you are no longer scared of death what is there?" The answer is even more simple: **Living!**

- If you want to fight against cancer that's great. Also fight against the apathy that occurs and is perpetuated by doctors who treat you like cattle and require you to quietly do as you are told. Start advocating for yourself and become an active participant in your own treatment. Yes, I know how scary, terrifying and exhausting cancer can be. However, if you don't become an active participant in your own treatment, you may feel even more lost and frustrated, feeling as if you have no control of your life or the direction you want it to take. I'm not advocating that you ignore your physician's advice. I'm challenging you to be a full participant in your cancer treatment. Question. Research. Learn.

- Never stop enjoying life to the fullest; merely be conscious of the consequences of your actions, and minimize risks whenever possible.

- Having cancer is like giving birth and showing all the baby pictures. At first, your friends and family are oohing and aahing. After a while, they get tired of the constant baby discussions — and really, who cares how many poopy diapers your baby goes through? Just like parents need a night out without talking about their new baby, cancer patients need time out without talking about their cancer. Designate a "No Cancer Day" and take some time away from your diagnosis — even if it's just for an hour. Do things you love to do or find new activities to enjoy. This will be great for you, your mental and emotional health, as well as your loved ones.

- **Question everything!**

- It's OK to be a little morbid and depressed at times. However, if you find yourself too often in this mood and unmotivated, speak with your physician, a social worker or a mental health practitioner. It's easy for breast cancer patients to fall into depression. The trick is not staying in that mood for long. Personally, I often go for a walk when I start feeling depressed or ill at ease. The walk not only helps me clear my mind, it is also great exercise and keeps me healthy.

- Angry days will come. You'll be angry at your doctors, angry at the cab driver, angry at God, angry at people on the streets, maybe even angry at the chair you sit in awaiting your next doctor's appointment. You'll even be angry and not have a reason for it. At times, it'll feel like your life isn't your own. Thus, find positive ways to feel in control.

     Plan activities designed to help you overcome this anger (depression turned inward). Find or create a foothold to get through these difficult days.

     It's perfectly normal; we all experience them.

     This is one of those days when taking a walk, playing hooky with the kids or a friend, or just being alone and sitting in silence will be good. Use the time for journaling;

excise your anger through writing. Get it all out. This will allow the positive thoughts to come in.

As Mike Dooley says, "Thoughts become things." Therefore, be cognizant of your thoughts. What you believe is what you will bring and create in your life.

Believe in the truth that there are more wonderful things heading your way. Sometimes, you just need to reach for them; to demand a little more from yourself, from your life, and those around you. It's never too late nor too early to start your post-cancer-surgery life. If not now, when?

• Let someone else do the worrying for you. Designate the worrier — your doctor, a friend or loved one. You enjoy life. Live to the fullest every day. Squeeze every drop of happiness you can.

• What would you say to someone who's going through your medical challenges? What do you wish people would say to you? Once you have it figured out, say the words to yourself. Better yet, put it on a T-shirt and wear it often.

• Be your own best advocate! Educate yourself on your condition and the resources available to you.

• Once a day, every day, remind yourself of your love, appreciate and gratitude for **yourself.** Yep, you! We often forget we need to hear those words from ourselves as well.

• The truth will set you free once you realize the lies that you've been telling *yourself* which hold you back from achieving your goals.

- **Get out of "survivor" mode and get back to thriving and living!**

- When you find yourself off course, merely redirect yourself!

- I will never lose the battle against cancer; I will, however, die one day, just like everyone else.

- Just do it! This should be one of your new mottos. That goes for everything life offers. Love. Sex. Adventure. New beginnings. The choices are yours to make — and the choices are wonderfully spectacular and endless.

- Indulge in bliss!

- It's acceptable to mourn the loss of your breasts, your hair, your life as it once was. Give yourself that respect — that permission. Then, move forward to create a new life, with a new self-image. Know that you can now create — not recreate but CREATE — the life you've always wanted to live. It's perfectly acceptable not to know what that new you will become. Merely be open to the possibilities. If not now, when?

- If you want to fight against cancer, fight against the apathy that occurs and is perpetuated by physicians and medical/health care providers. Fight against being treated like cattle and being expected to follow blindly. Fight against feeling helpless. Take control of your life. Become an active participant in your treatment, in your life. Yes, I know it's scary. Hell, it terrified me at times and made me mentally, physically and spiritually exhausted. Yet, if you don't fight and advocate for yourself, are you willing to accept the consequences? Misery. Despondency. Death. Choose, every day, and go from there. Don't worry if you fall — that's a given — just get up and try again; that's true courage!

- Indulge in bliss wherever you find it! (Yep, just had to remind you of this one twice.)

As you are discovering, there is a plethora of information and possibilities to learn, discover and discuss regarding your cancer diagnosis. Above is the information I thought was most important for you to know at this stage of your **Cancer Tamer Journey.** Yes, I purposely capitalize *Tamer* as that's the most important aspect to remember and keep in the forefront of your mind through this challenging time. You will *tame* the cancer within you. You will be as victorious as you wish to be.

Yes, you will stumble, fall, and rise again as many times as *you choose.*

Turn to others for assistance and a shoulder to lean on, even if that person is a stranger. I know I've fallen several times and contemplated giving up when the insanity of cancer drove me to my knees and the depths of despair. It's not pride that kept me here, nor was it merely the encouragement of others, it was that voice inside me that begged me not to give in. The same voice that begged me not to poison my body with chemotherapy. The same voice that declares, "I'll be healthy once more. I just have to be around to see it."

Always speak with your physician if you have any concerns regardless of how minor you feel they may be. These are your concerns. You are not whining nor overreacting when you do so. You are being a true advocate for yourself. Remember the old saying, "It's better to be safe than sorry." Discuss all your concerns with your physician(s). Write them down in your journal book along with questions that you want to discuss with them at your next appointment. You are entitled to have your concerns and fears addressed.

Ultimately, it is up to you to choose what's best for you. You must live for yourself, not just your kids or loved ones. That's the only choice that really matters when all is said and done.

Notes:

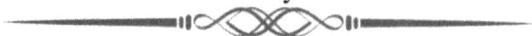

Notes:

CHAPTER 11

Preparing for Surgery

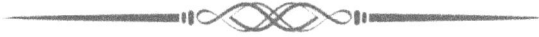

———— ❈ ————

You can never be *too prepared* for surgery!

The weeks before my surgery, I began planning and preparing to ensure I had everything I needed in place and at the ready. As a single woman with no family or friends around to help me during this health crisis — and admittedly unwanted cancer adventure — I was determined to be prepared as I went at it alone.

I cleaned the house.

Rearranged furniture.

Purchased lots and lots of sandwich bags and plastic containers so I could freeze my meals and have them ready to eat. (A few months after my diagnoses, I became very gung-ho about eating healthy. I went as far as tossing out all my delivery menus; even took the restaurants off my speed dial. Processed foods, fast food joints and sugary beverages were permanently off the menu.)

I cooked large batches of chili, even went so far as to pre-package shredded cheese so all I had to do was pull the packages from the freezer, toss them in the microwave and *Voila!* Food was served. Pretty smart, huh?

Wait, there's more. I got "green" fancy and made various healthy juices and froze them in ice cube trays, then placed the frozen cubes into more plastic baggies; this way all I'd have to do was toss the cubes into the blender with a little almond milk and, say it with me, "*Voila!* My nutritious delicious juice was ready."

I made enough combinations to enjoy at least two smoothies a day for a week. Perfect, right?

I was so proud! Even the medical staff and my friends were impressed.

I remember waking up in the early morning hours the day after my surgery, struggling to sit up in bed, holding onto my breasts as excruciating pain shot through me with every move I made. I was starving. Hadn't eaten in almost two days since they don't let you eat after midnight the day of your surgery. I braved the stairs down to the kitchen and stood before the refrigerator anticipating the feast within.

There was just one teensy tiny little catch none of us considered — not myself, my friends nor the medical staff. That's the fact that I would be **unable** to raise my arms high enough to reach the freezer compartment following surgery. Nor did we anticipate that the slight suction the fridge maintains to keep its door sealed and lock in the cool air would prove a challenge for me to open. I literally had no upper body strength after my lumpectomy and bilateral breast reconstruction.

And so, I stood there, in the dark, sobbing because I was starving, and my hunger merely compounded the pain in my chest, and worse yet, there was no one to help me which only served to make me more isolated and miserable.

I finally called the friend who'd brought me home from the hospital and asked her if she'd come over and open the fridge for me and help make me something to eat. She stated she'd be happy to help — in a few hours. I didn't realize it was

4:00 a.m. when I called. Besides, she couldn't leave her young son home alone merely to provide assistance.

As my cries died down to hiccups, I made my way back up the stairs, took the pain medicine she'd left on the bedside table and counted the minutes till she arrived at 7:45 a.m. to open the fridge for me and refill my glass of water.

We solved the problem with the suction seal on the refrigerator door; we left the door partially ajar so I didn't have to struggle and injure myself or tear my sutures since it would now easily pull it open.

Another thing none of us considered was the fact that I wouldn't be able to reach the top of my juicer machine to toss in the fruits and vegetables. I couldn't raise my arms high enough to dump in the ingredients. My only alternative was to toss the fruits and vegetables in the air, like I was playing basketball. I'll admit it right now; I'm no Michael Jorden. Most of the frozen cubes flew everywhere. I did, however, manage to toss in a few fruits and veggies into the blender which my friend had already filled with the required amount of almond milk. (Thank goodness almond milk doesn't spoil like cow milk does when left out.) Anyway, once everything was ready, I pushed the button, made my juice, and licked my lips anticipating how delicious it would taste.

You already know what's coming, don't you? Yep, that damn lifting problem. There was no way I could lift the pitcher. I was barely able to lift an 8-ounce bottle of water. Thank God for bendy straws. I just stuck the straw into the blender and sipped away. (Bendable or flexible straws are a major necessity during your recovery. Get yourself two bags full. They'll become a small blessing.)

You will discover that lifting anything, including water glasses, coffee cups, even small water bottles, will prove difficult. You've lifted these all your adult lives; yet breast surgery will make it excruciating. I recommend purchasing those small 8-ounce water bottles and placing one or two by your bed. Take the top off and place the bendy straw in it. Yes, unscrewing the tops may prove challenging as well.

Remember, your body will have undergone major surgery if you've had a lumpectomy or mastectomy — even if it's just on one side of your chest. Not to mention, the fact that you'll have tenderness and pain on your suture site and under your arm(s) where they removed your lymph nodes.

Don't be ashamed to ask for help nor make these simple preparations. Believe me, I would have praised anyone who would have shared these little tidbits with me.

Here's another helpful tidbit which I discovered the hard way. Pour your milk or juices into small baby bottles or into a small sugar jar. Those small 8-ounce plastic water bottles work great too. Anything larger or made from glass may prove difficult, if not impossible, to lift for a few days — even a week or more, depending on your surgery.

I discovered this little tidbit after one of my friends was sweet enough to bring me a 48-ounce jug of almond milk for my smoothies. She figured the bigger the better so I wouldn't run out of milk for the week. Neither of us realized I wouldn't be able to lift the jug. I will admit, there were a few moments when I was really jonesing for a smoothie and contemplated stabbing the jug with a knife and sticking a straw in it just so I could have something to drink. I won't admit that when I tried to do just that, the knife bounced off the plastic because I lacked the strength to even dent it. I also considered tipping the jug over and letting it spill onto the floor as I held a small glass under it. Luckily, my friend came over later that evening and poured the milk into small plastic water bottle containers which were more manageable.

It's OK to laugh at the weird situations you find yourself in. Granted, they may not be comical at the time; yet as you progress in your recovery, you'll chuckle at the insanity of the situations you will often found yourself in.

Before I share other helpful tidbits with you, I want to mention one last thing about preparing meals. Don't prepare large, "heavy" meals as your body may not be able to easily digest them, and they may not be appetizing. Think light meals like broths, chicken soup with small bites of chicken (not on the bone) or little plates of cheese, fruits, wild rice.

Heavier meals may not sit well in your stomach because of the anesthesia you're overcoming or the pain meds you'll receive. All that chili I made — which I make fabulous chili — had to wait for two weeks as even the thought of it was not appealing after surgery.

Below, I've listed several valuable points which will help you prepare for surgery and will come in useful immediately afterward. Though I'll go into further details in the second book, *Breast Cancer: From Surgery thru Treatment*, these tidbits will get you started and avoid unnecessary difficulties and hardships. I've listed them below in no particular order. You can check them off as you prepare yourself for surgery. I also mention a few to perform before leaving for the hospital.

- Some women like to "dress-up" for their surgery; this is perfectly normal. For instance, they'll have their hair done, their makeup done and a mani-pedi. Here are a few precautions to keep in mind when preparing for the day of surgery: don't wear any perfume. If you're having your nails done, be sure to have one or two fingers that have clear nail polish. This will allow the surgeon to check your blood flow/circulation. Your surgeon and hospital will have a list of dos and don'ts for you to follow.

- Consider carefully what clothing you wish to wear to your surgery. The ease in which you can put it on and take it off is essential. Wear only loose-fitting clothing, baggy sweets or yoga pants and large T-shirts; these are perfect. Flat shoes or slip-ons work best. Stockings, tights and jeans will be difficult to manipulate and should be avoided, if possible. Even if you aren't used to wearing dresses, consider wearing one that is easy to slip in and out of the day of surgery.

- You'll want to wear a loose blouse/T-shirt since you'll be sent home with bandages and a compression bra. You may even have drains which will add additional bulk to your chest. (Don't worry about bras. You won't be wearing one for a while other than the compression bras they give you.)

- As for underwear, it's up to you whether or not you wish to wear any. It's easier not to when you're in a dress. The reason I mention underwear is that you'll find it difficult and painful when using the toilet to push down or pull up your underwear. If you're used to sleeping in pajama pants, you may wish to forego them for the first week after surgery and opt for a long T-shirt or short nightgown. Use a comfortable summer dress around the house for a few days.

- Prepare your bed for your return from the hospital. Place new linen on the bed. Pull back the covers that you may easily slip beneath them. Have the pillows lined up along the middle of the bed to allow you to snuggle against them and keep you from trying to turn over. It'll be quite a few months before you'll be able to lay on your stomach. Even once you're able to, it will be a bit painful as your surgical scars will take months, even a year or so to heal. Keep in mind that though your suture area may heal quickly on the outside, it will take a bit longer for the inside of your body to catch up.

- Empty out your purse or better yet, purchase a small clutch bag that holds only your license, ID, phone and lipstick. Have only your house key and car key with you. In a few months, you can return to your full, "heavier" purse. However, you want to ensure you don't lift anything heavier than two or three pounds after surgery. (Your physician may impose other restrictions.) The main reason to avoid lifting after surgery is because you don't want to put stress on your sutures or irritate them which may cause delays and complications in your healing process, including tears of your sutures.

- Avoid carrying anything heavy on the arm where your lymph nodes were removed. Doing so can put you at risk for lymphedema. Lymphedema is an incurable disease associated with the removal of your lymph nodes which many women who've had breast cancer suffer from. I'll say it again, if you get lymphedema — it's with you forever and will adversely affect your quality of life! Something as simple as avoiding lifting with the arm where your lymph nodes were removed, will help protect you. Thus, if you carry your purse on that side of your body, simply switch sides or switch to a clutch purse for a few months post-surgery.

- If you live alone or have small children, you'll want to dress strategically as you may not have someone to help you in and out of your clothing, and you may decide to sleep in your clothes for the first day or so. Also, set aside two to three outfits that will be comfortable for you to wear and slip in and out of easily.

- Request your physician prescribe your pain and antibiotic medications a day or two prior to surgery. If they object, for whatever reason, DEMAND it. The last thing you want to do after surgery is make a run to the pharmacy to pick up your pain medication. You'll be sick and in pain. It's not time to drive around — which incidentally will cause you more pain, especially if you hit a pothole. Having your loved ones, family or friends run to the pharmacy to obtain it for you will require a sympathetic pharmacist. They'll have to present their ID, as well as yours, as your post-surgical meds will be deemed a "narcotic" or a "controlled substance." Even then, the pharmacy can refuse to allow your spouse, children or best friend to obtain them for you. And trust me, I say this from personal experience, Tylenol **will not** help with the pain; don't let the medical staff feed you that lie.

After you awaken from surgery, it'll feel like Freddy Kruger came to visit — and he'll visit you often in the first few days following your surgery.

If your physician refuses to provide your pain medication the day or two prior to surgery, speak with your pharmacist to prepare them for the situation. Don't just call — go in person. Talking to the store pharmacist and the pharmacy staff will make this situation much more manageable.

Inquire if the pharmacy delivers. Though this may be an option, if you're alone, you may not have the capacity to get out of bed or open the door and deal with the delivery boy. Thus, again, it's imperative to address this issue prior to surgery.

- If you live alone and have no support system or your support system is not available, ask your physician about being admitted overnight after your surgery. This is a matter of safety — yours! Prearrange this. Yes, your insurance will cover a night in the hospital, if your surgeon recommends it. If they refuse, and you do not feel safe to return home (and they kick you out as they did me), admit yourself into the Emergency Room and explain the situation to them. Note: As a surgical patient, you are more susceptible to infections. Explain your situation and your need to be segregated from other patients. You are entitled to be placed in a separate room and be seen immediately.

- It's essential to have someone pick you up after surgery. You won't be in any condition to drive, and even if you're not in pain, turning the steering wheel will be difficult and downright painful for a few weeks after. Not to mention, having the seatbelt tied across your chest may prove too painful to bear.

  Personally, I use the *Lymphedema Pillows Cancer Tamer* makes when I'm driving or am a passenger in the car. The *Lymphedema Pillow* creates a cushioned barrier between your chest and the seatbelt; you're still securely strapped in; however, it reduces the stress and pressure against your chest.

- Have a family member or friend present in the recovery room with you; this way, they can advocate for you when you're vulnerable, in pain and can't do so for yourself. I learned this particular lesson the hard way as I went to my first breast surgery alone, and the nurses who handled my post-surgical care were less than professional and downright criminal in their behavior. In short, the nurses literally grabbed me by the ankle and pulled me off the bed just hours after my lumpectomy and bilateral breast reconstruction. Yep, I had sutures from one side of my chest to the other. They even dressed me themselves and dumped me into a wheelchair despite the fact that I complained about extreme pain and nausea. My blood pressure at the time was extremely high, and I wasn't even capable of standing. The simple truth was the nurses wanted to go home and I'd already been there almost two hours after closing. And though I expressed my concerns, my symptoms, the excruciating pain I was experiencing, and the fact that I had no one at home to help, the nursing staff wanted me gone. Even my request to be admitted into the hospital for the night and the fact that I'd discussed it with my surgeon and my insurance company had approved it, fell on deaf ears. One nurse actually stated, *"There are sick people in the hospital. You're better off home alone."* Yet, the simple truth was they wanted me gone so they could go home. As I happened to be the only patient left on the ward that evening, there was no one to advocate for me and no one to halt their inappropriateness. The rest of what occurred is a story for another time as is the hospital's dismissal of my complaint. Their response to my complaint was to state they would be sure to speak with staff on better customer service. Thus, I hope my experience stresses my point that even if you're a loner, like me, this is the one day to allow yourself to lean on someone else, if for no other reason than to enjoy a great conversation and a few silly jokes before going under the knife.

- If you're single or have a limited support group, consider hiring someone to be in your home for the first two to three days post-surgery. They don't have to stay overnight or be with you all day as you'll tend to sleep most of the day away. However, you will need some assistance in preparing meals, taking your medicine and even taking care of basic hygiene. This is not only a necessity, it's a safety factor. If you're too uncomfortable with them helping you go to the toilet or showering, the aide can still help you walk to the bathroom and back.

- When hiring someone to stay with you, you can have them 24 hours a day or schedule them for two or three hours a day. It may be best to have them there in the morning and early evening (breakfast and dinner) as you'll sleep most of the time during the day for approximately a week following your surgery.

- Did I mention, you should prepare your bathroom for your return from the hospital as well? Be sure to have toilet paper handy — low where you don't have to stretch to reach; that towels are readily accessible, and that there are no tripping obstacles in your path. If you don't have one already, invest in a shower massager that has at least an 8-foot cord. Leave it hanging down for easy access; especially if you're short like me. You won't be able to wet your breast or sutures for the first seven to 10 days post-surgery, thus, having the shower hose will allow you to direct the water to the lower half of your body and attend to your intimate hygiene. Avoid tubs as getting up and out will prove difficult — even painful. Plus, you do not want to submerge your incision site for two weeks or more after surgery. Speak with your surgeon about this issue.

- If your friends or family can't spend the night, have them come early in the morning; 5:30 to 6:00 a.m. was the time my pain really kicked in most days. Provide them with a spare key so you don't have to get out of bed and answer the door. You definitely don't want to have to walk up and down a flight of stairs when you're groggy and in pain. If necessary or you're not comfortable giving out your house keys, you can always change the locks later in the weeks ahead.

- Be sure to speak with your insurance company about having a home health aide assigned to your case immediately or arrange for their nurse to visit you the day after your surgery so she can assign one. Unless you have a major *Cancer Tamer Posse*, don't let pride stand in the way of getting the help you need.

Yes, Medicaid and Medicare provide this service. Fight and demand if you have to. Sometimes your plastic surgeon (who's in charge of your case after surgery) will not recommend a home health aide unless you have drains put into your chest. They or their staff will state your insurance company will not pay for it unless you have the drains — that's NOT true! If he writes the prescription for the home visiting nurse to visit you IMMEDIATELY after surgery (not merely after the bandages are removed), your insurance company is required to send a nurse out. Surgeons are egotistical. They don't want anyone messing with their work. However, the home health aide is there to help you cope with daily life, daily hygiene, and when necessary, help you change your bandages to keep your wounds clean. Your safety trumps his ego.

- I HIGHLY RECOMMEND YOU INSIST — DEMAND a visiting nurse or wound care specialist to visit you once your bandages are removed. Though your surgeon may state that all you need to do is replace the gauze pads and empty the drains (which they'll teach you to do in the hospital before you leave), I'm a big believer in having a professional review my care. The visiting nurse or wound specialist is one more person to keep an eye out for any infections or other complications that may arise. (We will discuss these complications in more details in book two of the series, *Breast Cancer: From Surgery thru Treatment.*)

- Be sure to have plenty of cranberry juice and yogurt on hand after surgery to help combat yeast infections. Yes, it's an old "wife's remedy" and naturopathic remedy which typically works wonders. If you're prone to yeast infections when on antibiotics, speak with your physician about prescribing DiFlucan (or a similar medicine) with your antibiotics. Don't let your physician put you off about getting an over-the-counter yeast infection fighter like Monostat. That'll fall under the "Too Little Too Late" category. The last thing you want is to experience pain above and below. Talk about excruciating! (Yep, I'm talking from experience here and as one cancer patient to another.) Speak with your physician about this possibility before surgery.

- Another trick is to place your medication — antibiotics and those sanity-saving pain meds in a small dish or bowl next to the water bottle on your nightstand. Just one dose at a time so you can sleep through the night or afternoon and not have to worry about reading labels or opening child proof bottles when you're in pain and turning on the light is too much of an effort. (If you have small children in the home, you'll want to consider where to place your meds to keep your kids safe.)

- Prepare a few small plates with bite-size fruits, cheeses, meats and so on. Plain crackers are fabulous in case you can't stomach food and are still feeling a bit nauseous from the anesthesia. Yes, pain medication can also add to your nausea, make you groggy and unbalanced, even give you the shakes. If this happens, talk with your physician about switching to another pain medication. Sometimes, a patient can tolerate Vicodin (Hydrocodone) better than Percocet (Oxycodone) and vice versa. Again, speak with your physician about all your medication needs. I'm merely sharing what worked for me and my own personal experiences. Every patient is unique and has their own tolerance and reactions to medications. Getting a little food into you, especially some fruits and protein, will help you feel better faster. Don't forget to drink plenty of water to flush out the anesthesia and keep yourself hydrated during this time.

- Don't be afraid to ask for help and don't let your ego stand in the way of your health and safety. I thought I could do it all on my own, and I discovered, in a very harsh and painful way, I couldn't. Show yourself the love and respect you deserve and make arrangements to have someone available to help with your needs even if it's only for the first two to three days post-surgery at minimum — that's when it's most crucial.

When preparing for surgery, don't forget to consider your emotional and mental readiness as well. Speak with your hospital social worker or a therapist to help you address the major changes you'll experience in your life, both physically and emotionally. Discuss the way you feel and see yourself and your body. This is extremely important if you have reservations about the surgery, thoughts of death, or anxiety.

Personally, I thought I was going to die on the operating table. I discussed this fear with the palliative care supervisor whom I saw for stress management and meditation. I recall my discussion with him one day where I revealed my recurring thought of dying on the operating table. I shared with him that I thought I would die, but the doctors would be able to resuscitate me. When he confronted me about my comments, stating they were very negative, I explained that everyone in my family who had been diagnosed with cancer had died. I was taking a lot of fear and stress into that operating room with me — and living with it afterward.

Though the reality of my breast cancer will never change nor will the body modifications which came along with it, the way I address it and the way I live my life has, not only physically but mentally, emotionally and spiritually as well.

I did leave behind parts of myself — like my breasts. I left behind other parts of myself as well, like thoughts and behaviors that no longer served me; ideas that did not coincide with the way I wanted to live the rest of my life, past hurts which only added pain and were not constructive and much more.

Metaphorically perhaps, I did die on the table as the "Charley" I used to be isn't the "Charley" I am today. So much has changed in the months preceding my surgery and the months after it. I see life a bit differently now — as will you.

Thus, again metaphorically — or in reality — you too will leave behind parts of yourself. Consider releasing the pains of the past and the fears of the future and allow yourself to just live. To choose the new path you wish to live. To choose thoughts which will serve your future. To become nutritiously creative and walk for your health. The life you lead is a choice, one you make every day!

Thus, as you begin anew — following your surgery — start building the life you want to live and share with others. Don't cling to the past. It's perfectly acceptable to choose a new life, new health, new friends and make changes for the better. This may mean you must leave some dear friends behind or drag them along with you. As I previously stated, life is a choice.

What will you choose for yourself?

What do you want for the new life you'll live upon awakening?

Use the following pages to answer these questions. Also jot down a few ways you want to prepare for your surgery, whom you'd like present, and the clothes you wish to wear to help make this time in your *Cancer Tamer Journey* go smoother.

Notes:

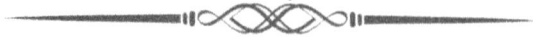

Notes:

CHAPTER 12

Emotional Health & Fatigue

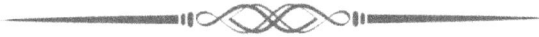

——————⫸⧂⫷——————

Fatigue is something that will happen to you regardless of how well you take care of yourself or prepare. It's your mind and body's way of saying, "I've had enough!"

It's inevitable that fatigue will strike sometime along your treatment and recovery, especially if you're undergoing chemo or radiation, have had any complications in your health or home life or get overwhelmed with life and all the Universe, God and the Goddess seem to be throwing your way.

Fatigue can occur physically, mentally, emotionally and spiritually. There's even a condition called *Decision Fatigue*, which is brought on by, yep, you guessed it, having to make too many decisions. Therefore, plan for it and prepare yourself ahead of time. This means creating your **Cancer Tamer Posse** and speaking to them honestly.

Your *Posse* should also include your hospital social worker and a psychologist, psychiatrist or therapist. You can also add your spiritual advisor or a healer you respect. Keep yourself healthy in all ways. It's OK and perfectly normal to lean on others when you need to. Don't worry, you'll be back to your strong "Wonder Woman" strength in no time.

Thus, prepare for these possibilities and have your support system in place. Though some people feel that discussing possible difficulties will make them happen, the opposite is actually true. It's akin to preparing for a storm. You don't wait till after the hurricane hits to board up the windows or stock up on freshwater and food supplies, do you? By discussing these fears, worries, or possibilities with those who can help and provide you with options (not merely sharing them with someone who'll listen), you'll be able to prepare for adversity and have the strength and tools to overcome it quicker.

Below are a few examples of ways to work through the various forms of fatigue and anxieties which will develop as you progress through this journey. Discuss these possibilities with your **Cancer Tamer Posse**, social worker, psychologist or therapist to help you prepare for all possibilities.

Mental Attitude:

There's nothing worse than a bad attitude. Like drugs, thoughts can poison your body. As Mike Dooley says, *"Thoughts become things."* What thoughts are you putting into your mind and how are they manifesting in your life?

Goals:

What are your plans for the future? What's on your *Bucket List?*

Meditation:

Meditation isn't just about sitting on the floor with your legs crossed like a pretzel. It's about taking a time-out from the stress of cancer, worries, kids, responsibilities, etc. and having a little "me" time. It's about allowing yourself to be selfish for a few moments each day.

I'm a bit too hyper to merely sit still and do guided meditation, and I'm not really coordinated enough for yoga so I do my meditation when I walk. I started out with walking the halls in my apartment building after surgery. Then walking half a block to get healthy. Now I walk three miles a day and use it not only as my meditation time but as my "healthy goal affirmation." (I do so dislike the word exercise.) During my walks, I don't answer my cell phone since it's my "quiet reflection time." I strive not to think of business; though I've been known to email myself on my smartphone with work possibilities before I turn it back off and continue my walk.

I love to walk in my neighborhood and discover all the amazing homes along the way. I'll admit, I've watched one too many DIY home improvement shows because I'll sometimes stop and evaluate a home and consider what colors, outdoor furniture or decors would look best.

When my aide or someone joins me on my walks, we can have discussions but mostly they are fun playful discussions about life and love and not focused on work or health issues. This walking meditation is how I relax; you may enjoy it as well.

Rest and Relaxation:

We often forget that after surgery our body needs a lot of rest to heal. Don't worry if you're sleeping 10 or more hours a day; you need it. If you're pre-surgery and you find it difficult to get out of bed or function, speak with your social worker or mental health practitioner about your lack of energy. Depression can cause you to feel exhausted and fatigued.

Exercise (Health Affirmation):

As I mentioned above, find something that you enjoy doing to help you stay or become healthy. Walking is low impact and you get to be outdoors. Yoga is fun. Aerobics or running is a great source of exercise; however, you won't be able to perform it comfortably for a few months after your surgery as you can tear your sutures if you're jumping around too much. Biking is another form of exercise. Find something that fits your style and personality.

Nutrition:

We discussed nutrition in-depth in our chapter on *Creative Nutrition*. However, just to reiterate, you can start eating healthy at any time. Yes, junk food and soda taste great; so do beer and wine and other things. However, if you're putting junk into your body, soon you'll be feeling like you're on your way to the junkyard.

One of the ways that I combat fatigue is by having an energizing juice or smoothie planned for myself each day and alternating drinks so that I don't get bored or rebellious. Starting the morning with an energy juice or smoothie sets the tone for the rest of the day. And, if you do get fatigued, at least it won't be "as severe" as it could be or those horrible sugar drops.

Just to be clear, when I mention energy drinks, I do not mean those over-the-counter shots or "sodas" that are full of sugar and steroids. I'm talking about healthy vegetables, proteins, fruits and nut drinks that you make in your blender or juicer. Remember cancer thrives on sugar, thus, avoid sugar products whenever possible and/or limit your intake.

Retail Therapy: (window shopping or actually buying)
I will admit I've become a true believer in *Retail Therapy!*

I used to hate going to the mall or shopping for items. My idea of shopping was one hour or less in a store. I'd grab what I needed and walk out. Now, when I'm feeling down or after a difficult biopsy or bad news, I'll go to the mall and flex my credit cards. And I've discovered the secret to healthy retail therapy that will keep you from going broke — only purchase goods from a store where you can return the merchandise with NO COST to you. If the store has a "no returns policy," don't shop there. You want to be able to return the merchandise when you "come back to your senses" and realize you don't really need nor want what you purchased.

Stay away from electronics unless you really need them and won't return them as most electronic stores will charge you a "restock/reshelf fee" when you return televisions, computers, record players, appliances, etc. Beware as some electronics will have a 7- to 14-day return policy. After that, it's yours permanently.

Keep in mind that some stores may have a "waiting period" of three to seven days before they'll allow you to return the items. Be sure to ask the store about their return policy and hold onto your receipt.

Now that we've discussed a few ways to overcome the various difficulties and challenges you may experience, jot down a few possibilities you feel will work best for you to overcome each one. There is no right or wrong in this. When in doubt or overwhelmed, discuss it with a trusted friend or healthcare professional. Feel free to share some of your thoughts with us on our website, **www.CancerTamer.org**.

Notes:

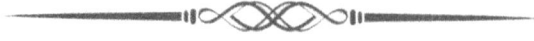

Notes:

CHAPTER 13

Resources
Organizations & Books

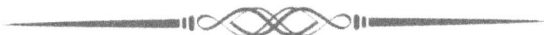

———————||∞⟨⟨✕⟩⟩∞||———————

Below is information on several organizations which provide services to cancer patients. By no means is it the complete list of organizations, merely those I know of and have worked with and found to provide exceptional service. I've also provided a list of a few books I've found inspirational as I travel along this path. On our website, you'll find additional resources and a fabulous PDF full of over 50 resources you can download which my dear friend and co-star on the Cancer Tamer Television Show, Debra Santulli-Barone, gathered for us. We'll continue to update this list on the website as we discover more, and you're welcomed to share a few of your own with us.

Organizations

American Cancer Society
www.cancer.org
The American Cancer Society provides education on various aspects of cancer treatment. They have trained operators

available 24/7, including holidays, to speak with you. I've always found their staff to be courteous, understanding and, most of all, knowledgeable. Best of all, they'll email you information on your diagnosis or send it to you in print free of charge. I will admit I've called them at various times in the wee hours of the morning when I was stressing about my diagnosis and had no one else to speak with. They also provide medical transportation through their *Road to Recovery* program. Though they have become a little too political in some of their practices, and many women's groups have protested their current stand on mammograms and other issues, they are still a tremendously valuable resource and have a wealth of information you do not want to miss. Contact them at 800-227-2345.

Bruce Lipton
www.brucelipton.com
Dr. Lipton is a world-renowned epigeneticist who provides valuable information about your genetics and dispels many of the old beliefs that "you are a victim of your genetics." His inspirational lectures and discussions will answer many questions and alleviate some of your fears as you discuss your genetics and your health care with your physicians.

Cancer & Careers
www.cancerandcareers.org
This non-profit organization provides conferences for cancer patients on how to work while living with cancer and information on your legal rights. They host conferences throughout the US, most of them free to cancer patients. Their workshops are fabulous and informative. It's also a great place to network and connect with other cancer patients who are working or returning to work.

Cancer Tamer Foundation
www.CancerTamerFoundation.org
This foundation is a non-profit 501(c)(3) organization dedicated to providing information to women (and men) who've been diagnosed with breast, thyroid and ovarian cancers as well as leukemia and other forms of this disease. We provide workshops and holistic care programs. We are raising funds to open our own **Quantum Healing Manor** where participants can explore holistic care such as yoga, meditation, reiki, sounds therapy, journaling for health and more. We also sponsor the *Cancer Tamer Television Talk Show* which can be viewed online. Visit us at link below to view many of our recorded shows. **www.cancertamer.org/list-of-shows**

Diva for a Day Foundation
www.divaforaday.org
Diva for a Day is a national 501(c)(3) nonprofit organization that offers women a day to escape the daily stresses they will face while dealing with cancer. They accept nominations from family and friends. One to two divas monthly enjoy a beautiful day of spa services at a participating salon. It's a fabulous day of rest, relaxation and a chance to restore your confidence and self-esteem. Contact them to learn more or if you're a spa owner or know of one in your area.

Dr. Charley Ferrer
www.DoctorCharley.com
Dr. Charley is a world-renowned clinical sexologist and award-winning author. She provides workshops on various topics, including sexuality, self-empowerment and preparing for breast cancer. She is the founder of *Cancer Tamer*. She is also the host of the Cancer Tamer Body Love Retreats. Check out our website for more information.

Gilda's Club
www.gildasclubnyc.org
This organization was founded by Gene Wilder in memory of his wife. It provides workshops and support groups for anyone impacted by cancer. The organization is based out of New York City and has offices in other states. Review the internet for a branch in your area.

Lipstick Angels
www.lipstickangels.org
Renata Helfman founded this amazing organization to help women feel gorgeous and proud of themselves and their beauty despite the ravages of cancer. Lipstick Angels works with various hospitals and provides a day of beauty to female cancer patients.

Rolling Thunder
www.rollingthunder1.com
This is a national organization that provides financial assistance to veterans and their families. I found their members to be very loving to veterans in financial need. Best of all, they actually host motorcycle road trips to raise funds. Look for them in your area and/or support one of their fundraising activities.

Stomp the Monster
www.stompthemonster.org
This organization provides financial assistance to cancer patients to help them pay for rent and other living expenses.

T.E.A.L. (Tell Every Amazing Lady)
www.tealwalk.org
This organization is dedicated toward helping women with ovarian cancer. This 501(c)(3) not-for-profit organization provides workshops and support groups for women with

ovarian cancer, caregivers and family members. It is based out of New York City and has sister organizations elsewhere. Check your area for them.

Thrive Market
http://bit.ly/2oOzrm7
Thrive Market is an online whole foods distributor who provides discount memberships to low income individuals and veterans. They are like a Costco which sells only holistic foods. Thrive Market has agreed to work with *Cancer Tamer* to provide our qualifying members with discount memberships and a possible stipend to use their services. Plus, they'll donate a portion of your membership fee to the Cancer Tamer Foundation. You don't have to be a cancer patient to sign up; everyone is welcomed.

Young Survivors Coalition
www.youngsurvival.org
This organization is focused on younger women with cancer. They also conduct the *Tour de Pink* bike riding fundraiser.

As I mentioned, these are but a few of the organizations I've worked with. You will want to research organizations in your area for emotional and financial support. Your hospital social worker should be able to provide you with information on local organizations.

My television co-star, Debra Santulli-Barone, was kind enough to research and provide an extensive list of additional resources which you can download in PDF file format from our website at: **www.CancerTamer.org/resources.**

Please feel free to share with us your own resource information that others may discover organizations in their area.

Books

Another great resource avenue is books. Below I share with you a few books I've found inspirational as I continue along this cancer journey. I'll continue to post books on our website and in our Breast Cancer Book Series as I find and review them. I'd love to hear from you about what books you find inspirational and a valuable resource. As ever, please feel free to post your recommendations on our website at **www.CancerTamer.org/books.**

Cancer: 50 Essential Things to Do by Greg Anderson
This book is both inspirational and informative. Within the first few pages you'll discover much about mindset and keeping your spirits up. What I loved most was Greg's way of inspiring you to advocate for yourself, and it's well worth mentioning. Just from the first 50 pages alone, it has provided valuable information and affirms beliefs I hold on treatment and other possibilities. I can't wait to get through the rest of it.

Crazy Sexy Cancer Tips by Kris Carr
This was the first book I read after being diagnosed with breast cancer. I found it very inspirational. It felt good to read about a woman with cancer who persevered and didn't let cancer "win" mentally. Her fun sassy attitude prompted me to purchase a few of her other books which you'll notice below and were a delight.

Crazy Sexy Juice by Kris Carr
This book is full of delicious recipes for juicing and drinking healthy smoothies. I loved all her juices and got to where I was drinking one or two a day. This is definitely a must-have if you're dedicated to living a healthier lifestyle. Best of all, you can tweak her recipes and invent your own scrumptiously healthy drinks.

Crazy Sexy Kitchen by Kris Carr and Chef Chad Sarno
I know these are quite a few books by Kris; however, she's well worth it. As a cancer patient herself, she has a unique understanding of what we face. Best of all, her recipes are fabulous. You can modify them to your particular tastes and, as always, use them as a stringboard to create your own. Be sure to share your recipes with us.

Biology of Belief: Unleashing the Power of Consciousness, Matter, and Miracles by Dr. Bruce Lipton
I loved this book. Dr. Lipton provided the information in laymen's terms with great analogies. No need to be a geneticist. The chapters on quantum physics and healing were inspiring. I wish Dr. Lipton would have written further on this topic; however, not to worry, you can catch his lectures on his website. I think the most crucial truth to gain from his book is the fact that you are **not** ruled by your genetics. You may have the genes for cancer or another illness; however, that does not mean you will be afflicted by that disease. You can discover ways to preemptively strike against it and keep yourself healthy, even go into remission. Check out his website **www.BruceLipton.com** and lectures on YouTube for more valuable information.

Breast Cancer: From Diagnosis to Surgery by Dr. Charley Ferrer
If you or a loved one have been diagnosed with breast cancer, this is a must-have resource book. It is a guide to help you navigate through the difficult-times ahead and prepare you for surgery. Dr. Charley provides personal insight on ways to make life run smoothly. Discover everything you SHOULD know but AREN'T told. This is the first in a three-part series on breast cancer, written by someone who's been in the trenches, endured multiple surgeries and complications, and advocates for the rights of women and cancer patients everywhere.

Radical Remission by Kelly Turner

This was truly an inspirational book to read. It provided information on what individuals were doing to help cure, stabilize or put their cancers into remission. It was also really inspiring to have the author address the fact that some cancer patients chose not to undergo the traditional treatments of cancer and radiation or discontinued their treatment and were actually thriving; not many books address this fact as it's a taboo subject in our medicine-driven society. The author also provides numerous stories of radial remission on her website: **www.RadicalRemission.com**.

Breast Cancer: Surgery thru Treatment by Dr. Charley Ferrer

If you wanted to learn the secrets of overcoming the ravishes of breast cancer to come out on top, this is a must-read book. This book is not about treatment options; it's about ways to cope with breast cancer, lead a healthier life to reclaim your life. Dr. Charley Ferrer provides valuable information and tidbits only other breast cancer survivors know. This book provides you with ways to thrive — not just survive!

Our book list will continue to grow in the months and years ahead. Feel free to visit our website for updates and to order your books or discover new ones. You can also download a free PDF with information on organizations dedicated to helping cancer patients. As ever, feel free to share your findings with us. **www.CancerTamer.org/books**

IN CLOSING

I know this is a difficult time for you. I hope *Breast Cancer: From Diagnosis to Surgery* has provided you with the information you need to help you transverse this challenging path. Though it may feel like it at times, you are not alone!

Join a few support groups, make tighter connections with friends and family and know that this is merely a stepping stone in your life.

Always look forward and imagine the possibilities. Though it may seem like you've just received your own personal *"expiration notice,"* it's not over until you're dead and buried. Thus, wipe away the tears, take the fear with you — since it won't go away — and decide to live your life to the fullest. Yes, I realize that sounds like the typical cliché, yet it's true. Better yet, try this motto; it's my personal favorite and one I endeavor to carry out daily, I've even scribbled it on the messenger bag I carry with me everywhere, "Live till you Die."

This motto isn't about death. It's about grasping onto life and experiencing every possibility, every moment you have on this earth.

There will be a pre-cancer you and a post-cancer you. Allow yourself to mourn the loss of your belief that you're immortal and will last "forever" and reach out to the truth that none of us knows how long we'll be on this earth. We can die in an instant or live till we're 113. It's what you do with your life that truly counts. It's the mark you leave upon this world through your work, your children, your family and friends, including the strangers you meet briefly.

I remember for the first few weeks after my diagnosis I would view everything as what I now call "the last time" syndrome. I got my hair done and cried as my beautician colored it as I thought it would be "the last time" I had a haircut and color. I cried as I flew to see my son across the country because I thought it would be "the last time" I'd ever see him again. I walked in the rain with no umbrella because I figured it might be "the last time" I'd be able to.

The beauty of "the last time" syndrome is the fact that you can flip it around from doom to adventure if you consider that it's "the first time" you noticed (perhaps in a long time) how much fun it was to walk in the rain and splash around in a water puddle, embracing the child within. Or thrill at the possibility of catching a snowflake on your tongue. Or better yet, getting out and doing a few of those items on your *Bucket List*. I've done all of mine; now I've created a new list, one which includes traveling to Machu Picchu and going hang gliding. Soon, I'll be able to say I actually "jumped off a cliff." Yep, I'll be soaring like a bird; how cool is that?

The world is full of possibilities--all you have to do is acknowledge them or **create them for yourself!** Become a *Cancer Tamer* and whip your cancer into submission. Discover how you can tame your cancer through creative nutrition, exercise, stress reduction, and rest.

What do you want on your *Bucket List?*
How will you live to the fullest?
If not now, when?

Live with *ROARING* passion,

Doctor Charley...

FUN & NAUGHTY
GAMES and ACTIVITIES

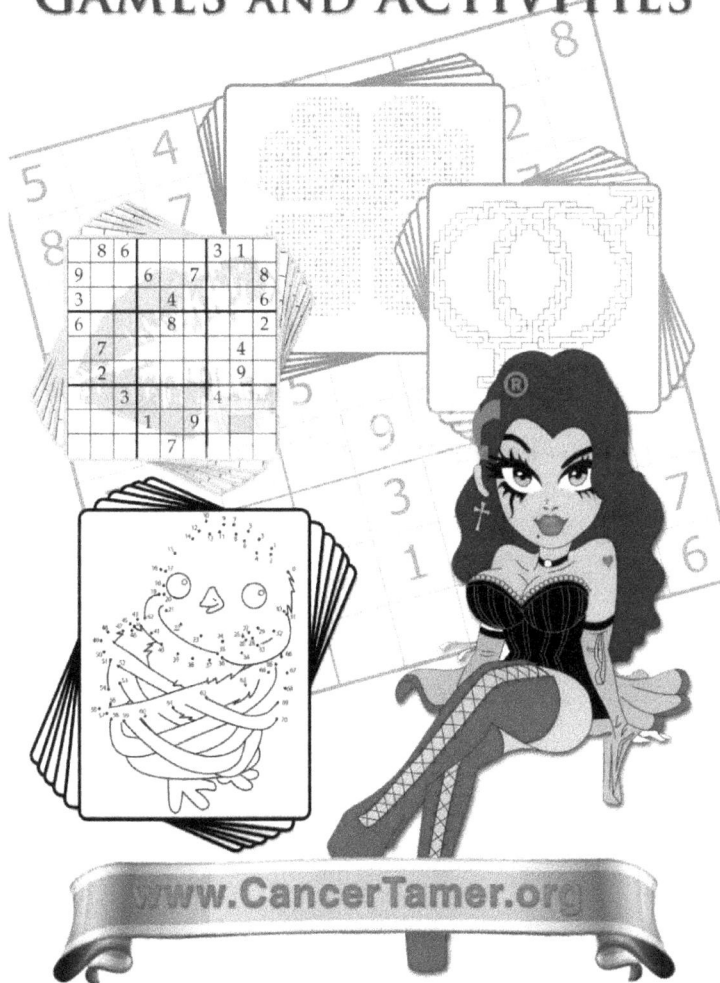

www.CancerTamer.org

Upcoming books by Dr. Charley Ferrer in this series

Breast Cancer
From Surgery thru Treatment
(Coming 2018)

Breast Cancer
Recovery & Beyond
(Coming 2019)

<u>BONUS</u>

Sex AFTER Cancer
(Coming soon!)

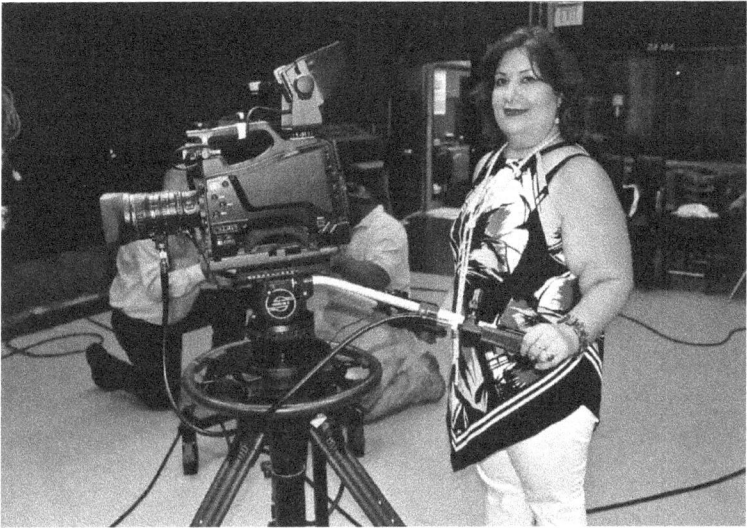

Dr. Charley Ferrer is a world-renowned Clinical Sexologist and award-winning author. For the past twenty years, she has lectured throughout the US, Latin America and China on sexual health and self-empowerment. After being diagnosed with breast cancer, she turned her fears and frustrations at the lack of medical information provided to cancer patients and the apathy they experience into a popular television series which provides information, education and inspiration to viewers. Wanting to help other women find the answers they need to thrive once more, she established the Cancer Tamer Foundation, a non-profit 501(c)(3) organization which provides cancer patients with services not readily available elsewhere. *Cancer Tamer* is a new voice for breast cancer patients! Dr. Charley also conducts various workshops and lectures on the down-to-earth uncensored truths about living with cancer and coming out on top. She is the host of the Cancer Tamer Body Love Retreats which provides a path for women to reclaim their sensual divinity and begin to love their bodies — scars and all — once more to enable them to embrace the life and love they desire.

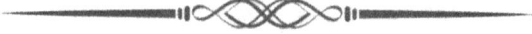

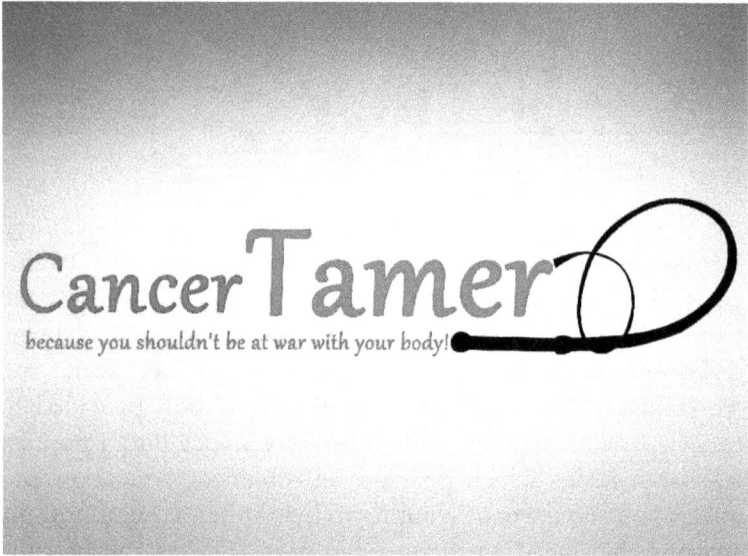